*Forgotten Leading Ladies
of the American Theatre*

FORGOTTEN LEADING LADIES OF THE AMERICAN THEATRE

*Lives of Eight Female Players, Playwrights,
Directors, Managers and Activists
of the Eighteenth, Nineteenth
and Early Twentieth Centuries*

by
Mary M. Turner

McFarland & Company, Inc., Publishers
Jefferson, North Carolina, and London

British Library Cataloguing-in-Publication data are available

Library of Congress Cataloguing-in-Publication Data

Turner, Mary M.
    Forgotten leading ladies of the American theatre : lives of eight
female players, playwrights, directors, managers, and activists of
the eighteenth, nineteenth, and early twentieth centuries / Mary M.
Turner.
        p.   cm.
    [Includes index.]
    Includes bibliographical references.
    ISBN 0-89950-453-1 (50# alk. paper) ∞
    1. Actresses—United States—Biography.   2. Women theatrical
producers and directors—United States—Biography.   3. Women
dramatists, American—Biography.   4. Women in the theater—United
States—History.   5. Theater—United States—History.   I. Title.
PN2285.T8   1990
792'.092'2—dc20
[B]   89-42759
                                                                        CIP

Manufactured in the United States of America

McFarland & Company, Inc., Publishers
    Box 611, Jefferson, North Carolina 28640

To my mother, Marjorie G. Turner

ACKNOWLEDGMENTS

I would like to thank the staffs of the Dover Public Library, the State Library of Delaware, and the Point Park College Library for their help in obtaining resource material. Aileen Elgie of Dover Public Library and Margie Stampahar of Point Park College were particularly helpful in tracking down inter-library loans of rare source books.

TABLE OF CONTENTS

DRAMATIS PERSONAE

CHARLOTTE CUSHMAN

MRS. JOHN DREW

MINNIE MADDERN FISKE

LAURA KEENE

FANNY KEMBLE

ANNA CORA MOWATT

SUSANNA HASWELL ROWSON

SOPHIA TURNER

"The Haunted Tree"

Dame Fortune is a fickle gypsy,
And always blind, and often tipsy
Sometimes for years and years together,
She'll bless you with the sunniest weather,
Bestowing honour, pudding, pence,
You can't imagine why or whence; —
Then in a moment — Presto, pass! —
Your joys are withered like the grass.

Winthrop Mackworth Praed
1802–39

PROLOGUE

*Every one familiar with the history of the theatre since it has had a
history, knows well, how great is the distinction between producer and
performer, and how few are the actors who have written clever plays,
how few the authors who have become distinguished as actors upon
the stage.*

— Laurence Hutton

The theatre is nearly as old as the human animal. Traditionally, man-
kind has ranked song, dance, tell-me-a-story, and spectacle just behind
food, shelter, and would-you-like-to-see-my-cave-drawings in the list of
basic necessities. When Thespis won the laurel-leaf crown in 534 B.C., his
art was already thousands of years old, and yet newly created with each performance. This body of tradition, combined with the excitement and possibilities of a live event, are what give the theatre its magic and its continuity.

Because the theatre has been remarkably free-thinking, women in the
profession have always been relatively equal to their male colleagues. Bad
managers have absconded with their salaries equally; audiences booed
them equally; they starved equally between engagements; and their contributions to the traditions of the theatre have been equally forgotten.

In the United States, during the last two centuries, the role of women
in the theatre was particularly ambiguous. On the one hand, the mores of
the times required them to be fragile, dependent beings, bowing to the
wishes of their male consorts. On the other, their profession required them
to be tough, independent, determined and strong-willed.

From the thousands of "daughters of Thespis" who "trod the boards"
from New York to Louisville to Sacramento, certain women stand out.
Their lives changed the face of the American theatre forever.

This book is about eight of those women, American by birth, adoption, or outlook, who have made remarkable contributions to the fabric
and tradition of the theatre in this country. Their names are hardly
household words, but each blazed a trail for those who would follow.

Selecting these particular women from the hundreds worthy of recognition was a difficult task. Of necessity, the number to be examined had to be

1

small, yet the sampling had to be representative of the diverse talents of the American actress. Each woman's role in the theatre had to be unique, and each had to be more than "just" a leading lady. It was possible to divide the accomplishments of the American woman in the theatre during the 18th and 19th centuries into four categories — actress, manager, playwright, and activist. There were numerous performers who fell into each of these divisions, yet from the dozens of candidates, the selection was narrowed to two in each classification. Each "leading lady" had to meet certain criteria.

The first of these was the nature of their part in the maturation of the American theatre. Any number of actresses in the 18th, 19th, and 20th centuries led interesting, tragic, or fascinating lives, but they returned little or nothing to the future of their profession. For example, Matilda Heron and Lotta Crabtree were remarkable figures whose stardom blazed and then flickered, and in the end they retreated into themselves and lived out the remainder of their lives in obscurity. Ultimately, they did nothing to enlarge or alter the history of the stage.

Secondly, each of the performers selected had to be original in their activities. In the past 200 years there have been innumerable actresses, playwrights, managers and others, but this book is confined only to those who were the *first* to embark on a particular aspect of that career. We are a nation which reveres pioneers, whether in space or the goldfields of California, and each groundbreaker somehow reaffirms the American spirit and the American mission. This is no less true in the theatre. The nature of the groundbreaking may be different, but the sense of adventure is nevertheless present.

Finally, each of these women had to be very much a part of her own century, and to be viewed in the context of her contemporaries. The theatre in the last centuries was very different from the modern creation with which we are familiar. Then, the theatre was a closed society, from within and without. It was as rare for an actress to leave her profession for "respectability" as it was for a "respectable" woman to take to the stage. True, there was a kind of tawdry glamor attached to performers, but like the circus tiger which would make a poor housecat, performers were thought best seen with a proscenium arch firmly separating them from the spectators.

Therefore, most actors and actresses tended to come from theatrical families and backgrounds, and this is true of about half of the women in this book. The rest took to the stage from financial embarrassment, fully conscious that by so doing, they were taking a desperate step — one that barred them forever from society's door.

Physically the theatre was very different too. Initially, there were four theatrical centers dotted down the East Coast, each serving as a hub for the companies based there as they followed a "circuit" of provincial performances. It was only after 1820 or later that New York began to dominate the American theatre scene, and the other regional centers — Boston, Philadelphia, and, to a lesser extent, Charleston — continued to be important for much of the 19th century.

Today, "New York" and "Broadway" are virtually synonomous with "theatre," and by "Broadway," the average person means 42nd and Broadway as the center of a roughly five-block circle which encompasses much of the "legitimate" theatre. It was not always so. For much of the period during which the subjects of this book were performing, theatre in New York was much farther south, in the area now known as Greenwich Village, and the neon jungle of Times Square was simply a pleasantly shaded greensward bisected by footpaths, perfectly charming for strollers. As "civilization" moved north, so did the theatre, until it reached its present location.

If the locales of the theatres were different, so too were the stages, and the techniques of the actors playing on them. Actors performed behind footlights, were illuminated by candles, and later by gas (which was harsh and crude), depended on their own voices to reach the topmost row of the last balcony, and performed with a formalized and stylized system of gesture and movement that would look very old-fashioned indeed today. They were surrounded with drops and side wings, or, later, box sets, all of which firmly grounded the settings and the actors in a confined space.

Unit settings, area lighting, platforms, moods "painted" with light, abstract scenery, and "conceptualized integrations of stylistic mechanisms" were as foreign to the 19th century as to Shakespeare. As it had been for centuries, theatre in America during the late 1700s, the 1800s, and the early 1900s, could ultimately be boiled down to a play and an audience, with actors in between.

This book is a study of eight exceptional, different, and very talented actresses who "stood between" the play and the audience. Each of the eight has been carefully chosen to reflect the growth in the sophistication and complexity of the American theatre, and the changing social and political forces in our history. Their lives enlarged and enriched the theatre and their fellow actors, and helped to create the "modern" American theatre.

Laura Keene challenged "the way it was done" in 1858 by heading her own dramatic troupe; her career was ruined by Lincoln's assassination. Susanna Rowson, twice shipwrecked, wheedled a pension for her father out of King George, wrote a novel that was a bestseller in England and America from 1797 to 1906, and was America's first female playwright. Mrs. John Drew, a star by the ripe age of seven, toured till she was 76, was the matriarch of the Barrymore dynasty, and ran the most respected repertory theatre in America for 30 years. Charlotte Cushman, whose ancestors preached the first sermon in America, began her career as a popular singer. After ruining her voice, she moved on to acting to become America's first international star. Many critics still proclaim her "our greatest actress." Fanny Kemble, scion of the distinguished Kemble acting clan of England, and niece of the great Siddons herself, married an American plantation owner. Her "diary of conscience" had an impact on the American Civil War second only to *Uncle Tom's Cabin*. Anna Cora Mowatt was a descendant of a signer of the Declaration of Independence. She eloped at 15 with a lawyer more than twice her age, and when he lost his fortune, recouped the family finances by going on the stage, and by writing a play, *Fashion*, which, 140 years later, is still immensely popular. Sophia Turner was the first actress to perform in the "West," establishing theatres in Pittsburgh, Cincinnati, and St. Louis, and overcoming enormous hardships to carry the theatre "west of the Alleghenies." Finally there was Minnie Maddern Fiske. Reared in the theatre, an actress from the age of three, she introduced Ibsen to the American stage, and was a "Trust-Buster," battling the absolute autocracy of the six men who controlled the theatre in the United States at the turn of the century.

These eight remarkable women were the first female playwrights, managers, actresses, and activists in the American theatre. They opened the doors for those who would follow, and created respectability where none had existed before. Their contributions were influential in shaping the theatre of their day, and the theatre that would come.

Unfortunately their deeds have outstripped their fame, and their names are now obscure. Yet rescuing from oblivion the first woman playwright or manager, however worthy, simply because she was the first, is merely academic. It is important to examine the impact each of these women have had on the theatre, if only to determine what the history of the profession might have been like without them. Each woman is clearly a product of her own time, and must be examined within the context of her century. In our era of women truck drivers and astronauts, it is less unusual for a woman to manage a theatre company than it was in 1865, when women were barred from voting and owning property in their own names. Twentieth century women manage companies, climb the Himalayas, and split the atom; in the early 1800s it was a daring soul indeed who embarked on the torturous journey of wagon, riverboat, cart, horseback, and foot to travel between performances in Cincinnati and St. Louis.

Therefore the lives of these actresses, which give us the background and context of their accomplishments, are as important as the accomplishments themselves, and are examined in depth so that the reader may gain a sense of the women as people, not as isolated "first" playwrights, "first" managers, etc., and, in so doing, realize how gigantic were their steps within the confined worlds of their profession and their centuries.

Act I

THE PLAYWRIGHTS

Aphra Behn was the first "modern" woman to write for the stage and when she began her career back in 1672, her attempts were viewed more as novelties than as serious dramatic endeavors.

The hundred years which elapsed between her productions and those of Susanna Haswell Rowson might have been 20 minutes were they gauged by attitude or the advances in the profession. Women playwrights were still novelties, much admired for their industry if not for their achievements.

Susanna Rowson made a career with her pen and her stint as a dramatist was only part of a long and diverse association with literature. Nonetheless, the fledgling American theatre, eager for nationalistic, and, above all, *new*, plays, avidly embraced the young woman with her facile pen. In today's terms we might see Susanna Rowson as a hack, writing to popular taste with no thought to posterity. She was a "commercial" playwright, rather than a "literary" one. Her successor, Anna Cora Mowatt, wrote purely from financial embarrassment, yet she elevated the stage and those associated with it to the genteel respectability which was her birthright.

Only one complete copy of a play by Susanna Haswell Rowson exists, and Anna Cora Mowatt wrote only one which has endured, but both left their imprint on the American theatre, adding respectability and resource to shape the role of the actress and playwrights for generations to come.

Susanna Haswell Rowson

The year was 1762. The royal regiment marched through the Portsmouth town square. Their light red "lobsterback" uniforms shone in the sun. Light streamed from their polished gunstocks and their boots glistened

5

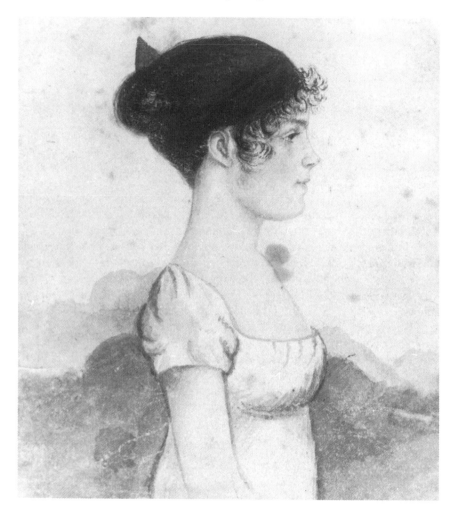

Watercolor portrait of Susanna Haswell Rowson (Susanna H. Rowson collection, Special Collections Dept., Clifton Waller Barrett Library, University of Virginia).

with oil. They were off to subdue the Indians in the American colonies. The afternoon smelled of excitement and leavetaking.

Lieutenant William Haswell's wife stood among the spectators, waving frantically. Her swollen belly and swollen ankles were the young soldier's legacy to her. When his unit marched out of town, he never looked back.

Soon after the soldiers sailed for the New World, his daughter was born. It was a prolonged, difficult labor. Susannah Musgrove Haswell lived only long enough to name her baby and entrust her to a nurse. The nurse was a good-hearted and resourceful woman. She had to be.

When Lieutenant Haswell was informed of his wife's death, he looked at his surroundings. America was a raw land with danger on every hand. The barracks were bare lumber and hard bunks and the officers' quarters were little better. The women who had followed the drum with their men were of two sorts—those brave enough and foolish enough to abandon the relative comforts of city homes, and those rougher women who cluster wherever there are soldiers.

Clearly it was no place for a motherless baby. Accordingly Haswell wrote to the nurse that "he would send for baby Susanna when conditions improved," and promptly settled down to the pleasures and hardships of a soldier's life. Five years later he remembered that he had a daughter.

In the interim, Haswell, who was handsome and charming, had remarried. His new bride, Rachel Woodward, was somewhat older than he and much wealthier. With the nuptials, he resigned his commission, and returned for his daughter. His standard of living had just taken a dramatic turn for the better.

He went back to England in 1766 to retrieve the child and booked return passage with Susanna and her nurse on a brig bound for Boston, sailing in October from Deal.[1] The rough stormy weather lengthened the voyage out of all hope or expectation. October passed. November slid by. December—the passengers celebrated Christmas by going on short rations of a sea biscuit and a cup of water a day. Ice hung from the shrouds, and gales swept the decks. The boat sailed endlessly in gray Atlantic waters, fog-veiled, storm-tossed, land-lost.

By the time young Susanna finally arrived in the city of Boston, she probably wished her father in perdition. During the voyage her nurse spent the time alternately clutching a bucket and moaning in her bunk. Evidently she was not a good sailor. The child explored the ship, made friends with the other passengers and the sailors, and speculated about her new home and unknown father and step-mother.

Finally on January 27, 1767, Boston Harbor was sighted. However, the harbor was not the end of the troubled passengers' stormy voyage. Outside Boston the ship foundered and Susanna and her sorely tried nurse spent three memorable, wet days in a cramped, leaky lifeboat, buffeted by waves and in constant fear of drowning.

Eventually a rescue party, led by stalwart ex–Lieutenant Haswell, reached them and the girl was off to a new life in America. The Haswells had settled in a valley outside Nantasket where their neighbors included the Otises, America's first family of letters and law. Mercy Otis Warren wrote *The Group*, a pro-revolutionary pamphlet set in dialogue form. She is often mistakenly called America's first woman playwright because of this, but her efforts were no more "plays" than Plato's *Dialogues* are.

James Otis, Mercy's brother, even then an *éminence grise* and acknowl-

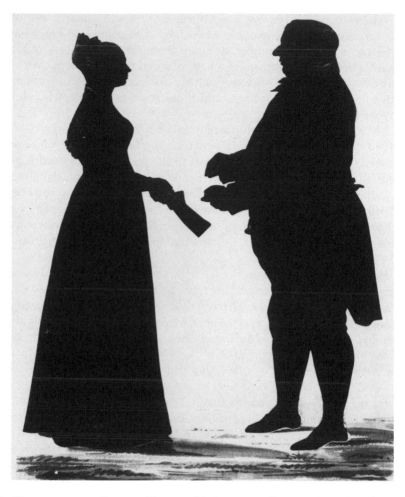

The Rowsons — cut silhouette (Susanna H. Rowson collection, Special Collections Dept., Clifton Waller Barrett Library, University of Virginia).

edged intellectual, took a fancy to Susanna and became her teacher.[2] Otis was one of the fiery agitators for the Revolution. He proposed the meeting of representatives from each colony which became known as "the Stamp-Act Congress." He was highly educated, a Harvard graduate, and for several years, King's advocate-general of the Vice-Admiralty Court of Boston. Under his guidance, Susanna moved from her numbers and letters to Greek and Latin. By her teens, she was reading Aristophanes, Euripides and Plautus in the original and relishing unexpurgated versions of Shakespeare and his fellow Elizabethan dramatists. It was a heady mix in an era when a girl was considered learned if she could read her prayerbook.

The Revolution broke out when Susanna was 16 and her world collapsed. Her father was unable to abandon the King in whose army he had served, or to disguise his Tory sympathies. Neither was calculated to endear him to firebrand acquaintances like Sam Adams, and he and his family were detained, removed from their home, and resettled miles to the north, preparatory to deportation. They lived in quasi-confinement for several years, ostracized by the community and ignored by fellow British sympathizers who questioned their loyalties as well. Both sides suspected Haswell of spying for the other.

There were battles nearby and a young soldier staggered into Susanna's garden late one afternoon. He died in her arms and she buried him under the squash that night, fearful that her father might be accused of murdering him if the body were found.[3]

Not long after this incident, the Haswells reached Nova Scotia and found a ship to carry them to England. Ironically this ship also wrecked and they were left with very little when they finally reached London.

Haswell petitioned the Crown for a pension based on his service to the King. It has been suggested that he was indeed a spy and that this pension was to be a consideration for his services. The British were very interested in James Otis' doings. It might have been very convenient to have an agent whose daughter was in and out of his home daily. Haswell's claims were at first denied.

Susanna took a position as a governess. Her employer might have been Georgina, Duchess of Devonshire[4] who was the patroness for Susanna's first novel, *Victoria.* There is no doubt that she knew the Duchess, but it is unlikely that she spent the next six months in France with that family. She was, however, employed abroad. When she returned there were vague rumors of an illicit romance, but no evidence survives.

Back in England, she found her father in near poverty, querulously awaiting his disputed pension. It soon became apparent that only the King could intercede. Susanna determined that he *should* intercede. Through the Duchess, she gained access to the court where she became involved with the Prince Regent, the future George IV. Prinny had an eye for a well-turned ankle and Susanna was a woman with a mission. She flirted and cozened, cajoled and promised, until, at last, the young roué signed the pension order. Then she danced out of reach finally and forever.

With her father provided for Susanna turned to her own future. At 20, she had tried being a governess and a courtesan, and neither career appealed to her. She was well-educated, thoroughly versed in Classical literature and the arts of the poets. She decided to write a "modern, moral tale."

Victoria, her first novel, was in the epistolary style, then rather fashionable. Susanna claimed, "The characters were taken from real life,"[5] and, as she would do in later novels, took as her theme the horrible consequences of straying from the paths of virtue. Nason, her biographer, says, "The plot is not very cleverly arranged; yet in some of the scenes we have an earnest of the success which the author was soon to achieve."[6] Her heroine "loves not wisely, but too well," loses her reason, is deserted, and suffers touchingly. The book had some success and Susanna felt that she had discovered her true profession.

Meanwhile she was indulging in her own true-life romance. Her father had retired to London to a house nearby a military garrison. The Royal Horse Guards were attended by a small band and since England was temporarily at peace, the band had little to do besides give an occasional concert. Susanna's fancy was taken by William Rowson, an aging, paunchy bandsman with impressive mustachios, and a resplendent uniform, who courted her with coronet flourishes.

After their marriage, Susanna came out of her musical dream to discover that she'd wed an alcoholic trumpeter who believed in *wifely* fidelity, but saw no reason to carry that precept so far as to interfere with his *own* pleasures.

Susanna saw that she'd made a major mistake, but decided that she had to live with her errors. While William cast about for an occupation, she wrote several more novels. The most popular was *Charlotte Temple*, a disjointed, sentimental story of a young girl's seduction and resultant degradation and abandonment and death. It was published by subscription, which was common then, and became enormously popular.

Charlotte Temple combined pathos and passion, love and loathing, morality and maudlin sentiment. It was the 18th century equivalent of *The Valley of the Dolls*, and Susanna soon found herself the author of a bestseller. Unfortunately the numbers and the profits were puny by modern standards. Since there were no copyright laws and "royalties" had yet to be invented, she received no benefits from the 200-plus editions of the book. *Charlotte Temple* is the first novel officially recognized as a "best-seller."[7] It was equally popular on both sides of the Atlantic and remained constantly in print from 1795 to 1906, selling thousands of copies each year! It has even been reissued twice since the Second World War.

Legends surround the book, the most persistent of which is that Charlotte Temple was a real young woman who was buried in Trinity Churchyard at the tip of Manhattan. As late as July 9, 1905, the *New York Times* devoted a full page spread to the story, with sketches of "Charlotte's" grave and the "true facts" of her life and death. The heroine was popularly supposed to be Charlotte Stanley, a connection of the Earl of Derby, and her seducer, John Montresor, was an exceedingly well-thought-of British military officer. Montresor was a relative of Susanna; indeed her youngest half-brother was named for him, and she was certain to have been familiar with the "family scandal" which surrounded the supposed seduction. Since one of her claims was always that her fiction was based on fact and that her true purpose was to write morally uplifting and instructive novels, we may accept that there is a possible nugget of truth in the story. Certainly, her readers believed it to be true. Many novelists claim that their characters "come to life" and take over the fiction which tells their story. Susanna's *Charlotte* may be said also to live. Long after Susanna Haswell Rowson was dust, the ephemeral and rather silly story she'd dashed off was read and wept over and cherished.

She followed *Charlotte* with several other cautionary tales, and as her readers had come to expect, they were sentimental, moral stories about young women thrown upon the world. She drew heavily on her own experiences for the episodes, and much of her own life story can be examined only in its fictionalized form. Despite the fact that her fiction was geared to the popular taste, one scholar who has made an extensive study of her work, Dorothy Weil, feels that

> [S]he aspired to be a serious writer and teacher as well as an influential force in promoting freedom for women. . . . Mrs. Rowson undertook nothing less than the complete education of the young female, religious, moral, emotional, intellecutal, and worldly. Her books are addressed to women, all her novels' protagonists are women, her subject is women; whether she is writing of the struggles of a fictional heroine, of biography, history . . . she addresses herself to themes important to the situation, education and rights of women. Working before the formal suffrage movement, at a time when only a few European or American writers had taken a strong stand in favor of female emancipation, she anticipated many of the questions that would be formulated by the later advocates."[8]

Perhaps some of her interest in the "situations, education and rights of women" arose from the unsatisfactory nature of her own marriage. Her biographers had suggested that the warning "Do not marry a fool; he is continually doing absurd and disagreeable things, for no other reason but to shew he dares do them," which prefaces her novel *Sarah*, is a direct reference to her own marital folly.[9]

William was proving to be far from adequate as a partner. In addition to his drunken infidelities he was a poor businessman. He tried the hardware business and soon failed at it. After an evaluation of their assets, Susanna and William decided that little was left for them to do but to go upon the stage, and in 1792–93, the Rowsons, together with William's sister Charlotte, were hired by Mrs. Esten of the Edinburgh Theatre[10] which is where they were performing when Thomas Wignell engaged their services. He employed William as prompter and Susanna and Charlotte for small roles in comedy and opera. Wignell, who was recruiting actors for his "New Theatre" company in Philadelphia, was an old hand at the business of theatre in America, and he desperately needed actors to round out his company and provide fresh faces for his audiences. As well as prompt, William could play the trumpet in the band, and act character roles and his wife, why, his wife could act too! She had other talents as well — she sang, played the harpsichord and guitar, and could improvise a song.[11]

Wignell was foolish enough to hire them. It was difficult to persuade excellent actors to forgo the comforts of home for the rigors of America, but even so, he must have had some qualms when his "company" gave their only performance in the Old World in Dover the night before they sailed. William, in his cups, was less than inspiring musically. Susanna, despite whatever theatrical exposure she'd gotten in Scotland, was plainly terrified. She was also difficult to hear. The other performers were even less effective.

The cast included a Drury Lane musician and his extremely fat wife, an embezzler from the Bank of Calcutta, a young "lady" of no "experience" and four gentlemen of good families who had never been on the stage before, but who accepted the offer as a lark. No one knows what prompted Wignell to make the offer in the first place. Subsequently the young men did very well as actors and one of them, John E. Harwood, married a granddaughter of Benjamin Franklin.

Wignell must have had a sleepless night pondering his mistakes. He decided that the long ocean voyage was his only chance to redeem his poor judgment. Crossing the Atlantic, he rehearsed them constantly, preparing the actors for their American debut. Susanna improved markedly, concentrating her excellent mind on the new career which William's improvident ebullience had marked out for them. Wignell drilled them relentlessly and under his stern tutelage, even William began to remember his lines and stagger less. In her spare moments Susanna continued to "scribble," and shortly after she arrived in America, a four-volume novel, *Trials of the Human Heart*, was published.

Clearly she had an ulterior motive. Charvat says that

> [S]he wished to exploit the market that absorbed *Charlotte Temple* is obvious from the plot of her first American novel, *Trials of the Human Heart* (1795). The heroine is the putative daughter of a man who tries to commit incest. Her parents die, her brother is a cad, her relatives conspire against her, she is cheated out of her inheritance, is lusted after by every male who lays eyes on her, is disappointed in love, marries a man she does not love, is wrecked in the English Channel, finds her real father and mother (a lady who at one time is wooed and won by the Sultan of Turkey without being subjected to improper advances), and is finally united with her real lover, now conveniently widowed. Subjected to every misery, she nevertheless gets through all perils (including a house of prostitution) unsullied.[12]

The company arrived in Philadelphia, much improved from Wignell's efforts. The yellow fever was raging in the city and Wignell removed them at once to Annapolis, Maryland, where Mr. and Mrs. Rowson and Charlotte Rowson made their debut. In Annapolis, one of the audience at a performance of *Othello* was so impressed with the "intelligence of the Moor" that he tried to purchase him from Wignell for five hundred dollars. Unfortunately the "sale" could not be transacted.[13]

The Rowsons remained with Wignell for the next two seasons, appearing in Philadelphia, Baltimore and Annapolis as the schedule dictated. Susanna was particularly well-received in comedy, vaudeville, and opera. Julian Mates, in his history of the early American musical stage, notes that "she helped the range of pantomime's interest by becoming the first female Harlequin in America."[14] In addition to appearing with Wignell, the Rowsons also played with Rickett's Circus, a favorite entertainment. There Susanna "danced hornpipes in the part of a sailor."[15] On stage she specialized in comic character parts including the Nurse in *Romeo and Juliet*, and

> [S]he was a *very good nurse*, and in every part, particularly that scene in which she goes to awaken Juliet. She displayed a thorough knowledge of her author and his subject. . . . I do not pretend to bring this lady forward as a first rate actress, but she is always perfect, and attentive to the business of the scene; . . . she has often come forward in parts of consequence, . . . and has always filled those parts with credit. . . .[16]

Mrs. Rowson's roles in Philadelphia included Audrey in *As You Like It*; Lady Bountiful in *Beaux Strategem*; Catherine in *Catherine and Petruchio*; Lucy in *The Rivals*; Lady Sneerwell in *School for Scandal* and Mistress Quickly in *The Merry Wives of Windsor*. She was warmly received by audiences and critics alike.[17]

Throughout the time Susanna was in Philadelphia, she continued to write and over the years of her association with the theatre created several stage pieces: *Slaves in Algiers*, a farce with music: *The Female Patriot; The Volunteers*, a musical entertainment based on the Whiskey Rebellion; *Americans in England*, and *The American Tar.*

"She began with some occasional lyrics for use in various plays and pantomimes at the Chestnut Street Theatre and from then on she was in constant demand as a song writer creating lyrics for such musicians as Reinagle, Hewitt, Van Hagen and Carr," wrote Julian Mates in *The American Musical Stage Before 1800*.[19]

It was as neither an actress nor a novelist that Susanna Rowson made her most important contributions during the 1790s. Once exposed to the practical necessities of the theatre, she combined them with the classical dramatists she'd begun reading under Otis' tutelage. The result was a fresh commercial product capitalizing on topical subjects, interspersed with songs and dances. The results were extremely popular.

Although her only interest was to improve the Rowson financial status, with the production of *Slaves of Algiers* she became not only the first woman playwright to be produced in America, but she may also be said to be the mother of that uniquely American art form — the Broadway musical!

The plot of *Slaves* ... centers around events on the Barbary Coast (modern day Libya). In the 1790s, Tripoli was the base for a fiery band of sea-roving brigands with a stranglehold on Mediterranean shipping. They exacted a price for allowing merchantmen to escape unscathed. One of their favorite targets was American ships and 15 vessels had been captured, and 180 American officers and seamen had been made slaves before the close of 1793.[20] The pirates arrogantly sent a demand to Congress for a payment before U.S. ships could sail in their territories. While the issue was debated, public interest was high and sentiment greatly favored "blowing the bastards out of the water."

Susanna Rowson's play loosely interpreted the situation and provided a young American hero, a sailor captured by pirates. He is befriended by the beautiful young harem girl and ultimately he escapes.... Susanna's history was skewed and her situation fantastic, but she provided a manly hero and a clever heroine in a tuneful three-act romp.[21] The public enjoyed the play immensely and even the political situation was resolved when Congress ringingly declared "Millions for Defense; Not One Cent for Tribute!" Susanna played the heroine, Olivia, herself in the first production at the New Theatre, Chestnut Street, Philadelphia, on the 30th of June, 1794. Ironically, when diplomatic relations with Tripoli were reestablished, America's consul was John Howard Payne, an ex-actor and playwright who had scored critical success in London in *Hamlet* — the first American actor to star in England. His play, *The Fall of Algiers*, was loosely based on an incident from the Rowson play,[22] but he is probably best remembered for the song "Home, Sweet Home" from his *Maid of Milan*. When he abandoned the stage for politics he established a precedent other actors have followed.

Susanna followed her success with another play, *The Female Patriot*, in 1794. This was an adaptation of Messenger's *Bondman* and was probably never printed. It was performed for the Rowsons' benefit on June 19, 1795.

"Mrs. Rowson's successful comedy of the previous season opened the way for a new comic opera from her pen, *The Volunteers*, a local skit of little merit," according to George L. Seilhamer in *A History of the American Theatre*.[23] With *The Volunteers*, she returned to current events to provide material for her dramatic pen. No copy of the libretto exists, and the only vocal score does not make clear the plot. In any case, the play was unpopular and probably performed only once or twice. It was produced at the New Theatre in Philadelphia in 1795.

The American Tar was the last of the plays she wrote for the Philadelphia company and when it was produced in 1796 all three Rowsons took parts. It seems to have been an adaptation from a play by Jacob Morton, but no copy survives to examine. The title suggests a return to ground she had explored with *Slaves* ... and, given the popularity of that piece, it is possible.

Despite the success she was having with writing for the stage, her domestic arrangements were continuing to deteriorate. William was drinking more heavily and becoming increasingly less discrete in his affairs. Eventually he went so far as to present Susanna with his illegitimate son, William, to raise. She took the boy and grew very fond of him until he was lost at sea some time after 1811. William was virtually unemployable upon the stage, but he was not fired outright, probably because his wife was a valuable member of the company. While Susanna's acting talents continued to increase, William's unreliability offset his considerable charm and Susanna realized that the theatre, a chancy living at best, was even more precarious in their case. Even her prolific writing was doing little to supplement their income.

Philadelphia had become rather too familiar with the Rowson family foibles, so she decided to return to what was, for her, home. Accordingly, in 1796 she and William left Wignell and Philadelphia and spent the season with the Federal Street Theatre in Boston: "[A]t the Boston Theatre she repeated many of her Philadelphia roles, but on the whole, enjoyed greater importance as an actress."[24]

In Boston, she continued to write, completing a comedy, *Americans in England*. She played Mrs. Ormsby in the first production in April 1797 and again when it was produced for her farewell benefit. As always there were roles for William and Charlotte. It was Susanna's last theatrical adventure. At the close of the season, she took her benefit and retired[25]: "In her few years upon the stage she had acted 129 different parts in 126 different productions. She and her husband had also appeared with Rickett's Circus."[26]

With her career as an actress behind her, she decided that it was time to put to use James Otis' teachings and pass them on to a new generation of pupils. "In Boston, in 1797, incredible as it may seem for a British woman with a somewhat disreputable husband and a career as an actress behind her, Mrs. Rowson opened her school for young ladies."[27] And, added Weil,

> Mrs. Rowson was singularly fitted for the office of a teacher. Her industry and intelligence were great and her knowledge and skill in household economy were almost unparalleled. Such were her accomplishments, her refined and moral principles, and her pious and charitable dispositions, that her friends were numerous, and her pupils represented the most respectable families of the community.[28]

Boston in the early years of the 19th century was working very hard to maintain its reputation as a staid, proper town with a blue-nose morality and little respect for "play-actresses." Only a few performances were permitted in Boston and these had to be of a "moral, improving nature." The city fathers were unenthusiastic about exposing the citizenry to the corruption of the stage. Their most scathing pronouncements were reserved for actresses whom they seemed to equate with harlots and streetwalkers.

This was the city in which Susanna Rowson, novelist, playwright, and actress, with an unconventional marital arrangement and a child of questionable parentage, proposed to open a select girls' boarding school. Amazingly, though she made no effort to disguise her background, she was successful in her new career. She began with one pupil, but in the space of three years, she had all the students she could handle. Her school became a haven for the city's elite with Boston's bluest bloods sending their daughters to Susanna Haswell Rowson, daughter of a deported Tory and a former actress, to be polished and educated for society. This acceptance may be a tribute to her final superb performances in a 24-hour-a-day role. It may have been difficult for her to give up the enjoyable life of the theatre,

> . . . but by then she had come to realize that her peculiar combination of talents—literary, dramatic, and musical—might fit her for the less precarious career of school teacher. . . . She introduced the piano in place of the harpsichord, engaged a professor of languages, taught her students to recite long declamatory poems, and instructed them in social conversation and good manners. She . . . personally led them in the latest dance steps.[29]

William also found a home in Boston's pubs and he remained amicably in the city, occasionally visiting his wife to improve upon his allowance or to entertain the girls at an impromptu musicale. In 1802 he became a citizen and received a sinecure of a job in the Boston customs house. Susanna Rowson, model of rectitude, was never impervious to his charm, and she welcomed his visits, but they led increasingly separate lives. After her death, he remarried Hannah Bancroft and faded from the record of history.

The only remnant of the old Susanna which she permitted to exist, was her devotion to her pen. Just as it had been all her adult life, her writing was her solace, her avocation, and her source of extra income. Charvat provides a dispassionate assessment of her abilities as an author.

> She was a born teacher with a strong itch to write. . . . As a schoolmistress she had an occupation which served her as a patron while she produced verse, non-sensational domestic fiction, magazine miscellanea, and textbooks for children. She was the same highly moral woman that she had been while she was writing Richardsonian soap opera for Lane in England, and felt not at all ashamed of her past as an actress or a Minerva novelist. But the conditions of book distribution and reader patronage were different here, and Mrs. Rowson adapted to them without fussing.
>
> This readiness to consult the market and adapt to it her literary stock-in-trade, which was didacticism, gives Mrs. Rowson standing as an early American writer of true professional temperament.[30]

Now that she was no longer associated with the theatre, Susanna abandoned her playwriting. Her market outlet had dried up and she was not so enamored of the theatre as to continue to write for it on an "amateur" basis. Then too, in her newly respectable role as a schoolmistress, writing plays for production would have been slightly scandalous and would have undermined her hard-won social standing. However, *Slaves in Algiers* remained popular for some time after she left the stage. She continued to produce novels, now even more moral and improving than before, but the main thrust of her one-woman book factory was textbooks. She wrote a series of books, at first only for the use of her own students, but they were so excellent and there was such a dearth of similar material, that they were soon published and used all over the Northeast for 50 years or more. They covered a variety of subjects — reading, geography, deportment, mathematics, literature, elocution and science. In addition, her students presented a performance every year, of poetry and songs, and these too were from her ready pen. She rehearsed the girls in their presentations so that they made a graceful and professional appearance. Her young ladies were well-educated, polished, graceful and charming, ready to enter society with conversation and accomplishments, rather than simpers and silences. Parents, viewing the results, ignored the rumors about her past and flocked to place their girls under her tutelage: "Many of them are now to be seen in the refined and polished circles of the capital of New England."[31]

Susanna remained in the Boston area for the rest of her life, devoting herself to her students and her school. Gradually her past faded to sepia-toned memories as the girl who had flirted with and flummoxed George IV, and who charmed audiences with her acting and roused them with her plays, was transformed into a stern preceptress and educator. It was a role with which she was particularly comfortable. Her school prospered, and in time, few in Boston could believe that she had ever enjoyed the notoriety of the stage.

Music remained one of her pleasures and was emphasized in her curriculum. She owned one of the first pianos in the country, and her school was the first to offer instruction in this new instrument which was replacing the spinet and the harpsichord. Among the instructors whom she employed were Peter von Hagen and Gotlieb Graupner, "the father of American orchestral music,"[32] both of whom later became famous as music publishers and composers. Graupner also collaborated with Susanna on numerous songs which were published. He supplied the music and she the lyrics. The Graupners were old friends of hers with whom she had played during her season at the Federal Street Theatre. "The Graupner and Rowson families were always on intimate terms with each other [and] They occupied the same pew in Dr. John S.J. Gardiner's Church."[33]

Susanna moved her school several times as it outgrew its quarters, eventually ending up on Hollis Street in Boston. After ill health forced her to give up active participation in school affairs, it was taken over by her adopted daughter Fanny Mills, and her nieces Susan Johnston and Rebecca

Cordis Haswell. It had become "one of the most famous girls schools in America"[34] and its owner one of the most respected literary women in Boston. During the quarter of a century when she was an educator, Susanna Rowson edited one magazine, wrote voluminously for others, including essays, poetry and songs, created numerous textbooks and novels, and assumed leadership of several charitable organizations. Evidently she was incapable of wasting a single moment.

Nevertheless, when she died on March 24, 1824, her legacy was scant. She was beloved by her former pupils and her friends, although vitually ignored by her husband. "She died . . . respected, beloved, and regretted by all who knew her,"[35] and "was entombed . . . in the family vault, No. 14, of her friend Mr. Gotlieb Graupner, beneath St. Matthew's Church, South Boston."[36]

She left no direct descendants and only the literary works she had created survived her. Not all of them can be considered fitting memorials. Her novels were sentimental and romantic, and though they remained heavy sellers, they were not great literature. However, Charvat contends," Mrs. Susanna Rowson . . . is entitled to consideration as the first American professional writer of fiction."[37] She created "the misery novel"[38] which has, over the centuries, been transformed into the "bodice-rippers" so recently popular in mainstream fiction. It is a tribute of sorts, perhaps, to have written a novel, *Charlotte Temple*, which has outlived its author and generations of readers and virtually singlehandedly to have created an entire genre of fiction, even if it is neither scholarly nor literary.

Her textbooks were used for several decades after her death and then discarded, hopelessly out-of-date. Her plays were the relics of a different era, and by 1824, they had fallen into obscurity and were rarely produced. All have virtually disappeared, and today a copy of any of them is a curiosity, and a bibliophile's dream. The fragments which do survive are incomplete and deceptive. It is difficult to obtain any true sense of Susanna's real dramatic talents from them. However, it is the *fact* of her accomplishments rather than the deeds themselves which has become important.

Susanna Haswell Rowson paved the way for the women who would follow her—playwrights like Anna Cora Mowatt, Edna Ferber, and Beth Henley. Their success was, in some measure, possible because she created her own, and demonstrated that gender has little to do with the talents of the pen. Women could be as successful in the drama as their male colleagues.

Her novels survived into the 20th century, but were eventually put aside. Her position as a pioneer of the stage and as the first American woman playwright can never be superseded. It is a permanent memorial.

Anna Cora Mowatt

With trembling fingers, 15-year-old Anna Ogden unpinned a sprig of white geranium from her hair. She smoothed her best dress and looked once more around her room. It had been sanctuary, pirate deck, cave, and island paradise — all in her imagination. She touched the small rocker. She had spent many rainy Saturdays curled here with a book or a volume of Shakespeare's plays, planning the next family theatrical. No one questioned her right to play all the leading roles *and* order all the others around beside. From the superiority of "almost sixteen" she shook her head over her 12-year-old Lady Macbeth. "Oh, the folly of youth," she thought and picked up her cloak from her bed. She grasped a small portmanteau and slipped out, carefully avoiding her brothers and sisters. She went to meet James Mowatt, the 30-year-old lawyer, she'd married the day before.

When word of the elopement reached her parents that evening, Anna Cora's mother wept a little for the loss of her daughter's girlhood, and, finding that geranium branch, stuck it in a little water where it rooted and grew.

Like the plant, Anna Cora's precocious marriage was hearty and healthy, and her husband nurtured her as tenderly as her mother cared for the geranium. During the next three years, she studied languages, art, music, and literature under his instruction and thrived in the big house he'd bought for her pleasure.

She was the daughter of Samuel Ogden and Eliza Lewis, the granddaughter of a noted Episcopalian bishop and the great-granddaughter of Francis Lewis, a signer of the Declaration of Independence. Her father was a man of business and adventure who financed an abortive South American revolution, nearly involving America in an unwanted war with Spain, and who made and lost at least two fortunes. Anna Cora was born in France in 1819 when the family lived there while her father was recouping his losses. She was the ninth of fourteen children born to his first wife, Eliza Lewis Ogden. Eliza was a patient mother, as indeed she must have had to have been, but also a very determined one as well. She resolved to live to the age of 50, and died months after her fiftieth birthday — to the great distress of her family.

The Ogdens' return from France, when Anna Cora was five, was a disaster. The first ship on which they sailed met high seas and a great storm and two of the Ogden boys were swept from the deck. Gabriel was lost forever, but Thomas seized a piece of rope and was rescued. The ship limped back to port. The second attempt at a crossing was less arduous and Anna Cora returned to a native land she'd never seen, whose language she did not speak. With the resiliency of youth she quickly adapted, and, always precocious, plunged into schooling. Her progress was uneven. Even though she'd spoken French all her life, its grammar was a mystery and numbers simply dismayed her. At literature and writing, however, she was always first in her class. She read a great deal, and not surprisingly, when time for her elopement arrived, she behaved in a most romantic fashion, straight out of one of her favorite novels. She and her sister pawned their jewelry to buy bridal clothes, enlisted the aid of a nurserymaid to carry out their schemes, and hid their purchases at a shop on the corner until they could be smuggled, piecemeal, into the house. It was all most thrilling and very like the more lurid fiction of the time.

Her letter telling of her marriage was badly received by her father, who disowned her and threatened her husband. After three days of tears and endless letters, he relented in the best fictional tradition, and a reconciliation was effected.

James Mowatt did not expect his child-bride to keep house so he hired a housekeeper and saw to his wife's development instead. What should have been a ruinous marriage was a happy and productive one, marked by love and respect. Like a storybook, the ending was happy!

Under his care, Anna Cora cultivated her mind. She had always had an interest in writing and now began in earnest, aided by the atmosphere of Melrose, the house which they rented and later bought. James indulged her every whim as he watched his "Lily" grow to womanhood. For her part Anna Cora was devoted to him.

At 17, she began to write an epic, *Pelayo or the Caverns of Cavadonga*, a political romance in five cantos. She applied herself assiduously to her labors by day and read the results aloud to James at night. He was entranced and she was learning to use her voice to sway an audience.

The poem was published in 1836 to almost universal critical disdain. Anna Cora replied with *Reviewers Reviewed*, a satire on the critics who seemed to dislike *Pelayo* mostly because it was by an American author, rather than because it was a fairly dreadful and vastly overwritten juvenile work. *Reviewers Reviewed* was somewhat better received, but the whole matter was soon put behind her, and she and her sisters resumed their amateur family theatricals — now called "Concerts" and presented weekly.

In 1837 this idyllic life was interrupted when Anna Cora contracted bronchitis and was sent abroad with an aunt to recuperate. From England, the ladies ventured to the Continent. James was able to join them in early January in Germany. His appearance — four weeks early — had an unfortunate result. His wife jumped up from the piano at the sight of him and suffered a hemorrhage of the lungs, thus delaying their reunion by several days. She was to be troubled by weakness in her chest the rest of her life. Doctors thought it the result of the drenching she'd undergone on the voyage on which her brother drowned.

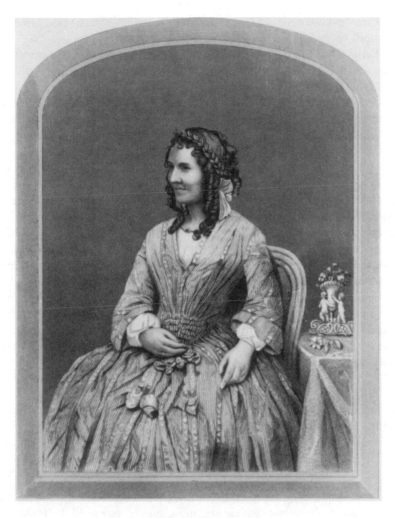

Anna Cora Mowatt

While they were in Bremen, James suffered an attack of a virulent eye disease. For several months he could only sit in a darkened room while suffering excruciating pain. They went to Paris to consult Dr. Hahnemann, the famous homeopathic surgeon. The trip was exhausting, and James was too ill to go to the doctor's office, while the 85-year-old Hahnemann was too old to leave his quarters. Finally a curious compromise was reached. Anna Cora went to Hahnemann's office where she described James' symptoms to the doctor's wife who acted as his assistant. Not surprisingly, James did not improve. He had resigned himself to a life of blackened rooms and pain when an American surgeon, on vacation, agreed to look at the son-in-law of his old friend Samuel Ogden. Within weeks, James was able both to stroll and to see the streets of Paris.

Relieved of the worry of her husband's illness, Anna Cora entered the social whirl of Paris, attending the theatre nightly and writing daily. Her efforts this time produced *Gulzara, or The Persian Slave*, a drama in six (!) acts. When the Mowatts sailed for home, their luggage included elaborate scenery. *Gulzara* was to be performed at their homecoming in a magnificent family extravaganza.

They didn't know it then, but this was to be the last grand social occasion at "Melrose." James' eyes were better, but not up to the strain of resuming his law practice with all the consequent reading involved. He began to speculate. At first all went well, and he made money; then came the currency crisis, and the subsequent financial panic. In weeks he was ruined, his substantial fortune swept away. His hardest chore was telling Anna Cora that her beloved "Melrose" was hers no longer. After the initial panic and shock wore off, Anna Cora began to cast about for ways to ease their financial woes. Soon she remembered that *Gulzara* had been well received and that Epes Sargent had even solicited its publication. Perhaps this way might lead to salvation. In fact, why not take matters a step further and offer public readings of the recitations that had so pleased her family and friends.

Her sister Mary was appalled and tearfully begged her not to expose herself to the public:

"But you will lose your place in society."

"If I fail . . . probably I shall; but I do not intend to fail."[1]

James fell in with her plan and Anna Cora followed her resolve to Boston. Promotional copy for her recital announced:

> Mrs. Mowatt's Recitations—The public are invited . . . to an entertainment of a somewhat novel character . . . its adaptations to gratify a refined taste. It consists of readings and recitations in poetry, with introductory remarks upon the perspective pieces, by a lady who is most respectably recommended, for her eminent literary accomplishments, and for those accomplishments which are most highly esteemed in fashionable society . . ."[2]

Despite weeks of rehearsal and years of private performances, she was almost overcome by stage fright. A last minute letter of encouragement from her father, and an uplifting visit from a Boston friend, sent her out into the hall determined to conquer adversity and Boston. By the end of the evening she had completely succeeded:

> Her first reading was given at the Mason's Temple on Thursday evening, October 28, 1841. She carried with her the heart of every listener for she exhibited the most beautiful moral spectacle of which human nature is capable, that of a wife turning her accomplishments to account to relieve the necessities of her husband.[3]

The Boston public took her completely to their hearts and the houses were packed. Local papers sang her praises unreservedly. Anna Cora was a success:

> Her Youth and Beauty, though sufficient of themselves to command attention were lost sight of when she began to speak, and one had the leisure only to regard the exquisite tones of her voice as it gave utterance to her admirable conceptions of poetical genius. Her stay in this city was brief, but the judgement then pronounced upon her abilities was final, for having passed through the ordeal of Boston criticism, and met with approval, she fearlessly went forth to fascinate by the loveliness of her person, and to captivate by the genuineness of her talent.[4]

She determined to brave New York, for until she had success there, she could not be sure that she'd chosen the right course. En route, she played a one-night stand in Providence, where a member of the audience was driven to hysteria by the pathos of Anna Cora's recitation of the poem on the destruction of the ship *President*, which had been written for her by Epes Sargent.

New York was much more difficult. Her erstwhile friends attended the first series at Stuyvesant Hall, condemning far more than they praised. Their scorn was not for the merits of her performance. Rather, the mere fact that she and James had chosen to support themselves this way, caused the less generous of their acquaintances to villify them.

The crowds still came to Anna Cora's readings, but the atmosphere was different. Where Boston had seen a gallant young woman defending her own, and seeking independence, New York saw an impudent hussy defying her class and her station to display herself. Anna Cora was determined to carry on. Throughout, James' only concern had been for her always precarious health, and, chilled by her reception, as well as the New York winter, this finally betrayed her. In 1842, she fell prey to galloping consumption. The disease was nearly always fatal and even the doctor who had rescued James' vision could offer little hope for Anna Cora.

Finally, she was placed in the hands of a physician who was also a practicing mesmerist. In those days mesmerism was believed to heal as well as delve into the Beyond, and Dr. Channing proposed to heal her with this metaphysical medicine. Anna Cora was reluctant to surrender her will at first, but her coughing fits were increasingly violent and there was no doubt that she might die. From the first the trances were almost miraculously effective. In the trance state, Anna Cora did not cough and she awoke from each session more improved until she was being touted as a medical mesmeristic phenomenon. Epes Sargent, who assisted in the trances, once left her in the trance-state for two weeks during a violent relapse. When he and James took her out, they covered her face with a heavy veil so that her rolled-up eyes and stare, common to a trance, would not be commented upon.

Anna Cora and James spent the summer in the country and when they returned, she intended to resume her recitations. However, she was not strong enough to sustain public performances and looked for another method of employment. Women's magazines were beginning to become popular, and during the summer she'd met a young lady who earned her living by writing for them.

In short order, Anna Cora was producing a steady stream of nonfiction and fiction ranging from "Bridal Customs of Germany" to a prize-winning novel, *The Fortune Hunters*. Under contract to a publisher she wrote a variety of books geared to the housewife in her practice of domestic economy. *Etiquette of the Toilette, Housekeeping Made Easy, Knitting, Netting and Crochet*, et al., were among her more popular titles, and, given Anna Cora's limited exposure to all matters of housekeeping, this must be regarded as a tribute to her clear writing style and the general dearth of available competing material.

James formed Mowatt and Co., Publishers, and Anna Cora wrote for his publication a *Life of Goethe* and *The Memoirs of Mme. D'Arblay*. These were far from best sellers and she was forced to return to the domestic front, turning out *Etiquette of Marriage* and *Management of the Sickroom*. Like most of her output to date, these were produced pseudonymously (*Sickroom* was by "Dr. Charles Lee, M.D.")

By careful management of her time and studious concentration on the demands of her public, Mowatt and Co. flourished. Epes Sargent also wrote for James, and established *Modern Standard Drama*, later taken over by Samuel French. This is the major source of 19th century plays.

During 1842–45, Anna Cora Mowatt wrote at least 11 nonfiction books, a number of articles, uncounted poems, the immortal *Fashion* ("the most important play written by an American up to that time"[5]), and two novels including the two-volume *Evelina* which was a tremendous success when it appeared, following *Fashion's* debut.

During this time, she also adopted three children, Margaret, John, and William Gray, the offspring of impoverished English immigrants. She had had no children during the ten years of her marriage, a fact which Eric Barnes, her major biographer, attributed to unexplained marital omissions and the illnesses of both parties, suggesting that the passion channeled into her performances was drawn from unexplored moments in the bedroom.[6]

In 1845, Anna Cora, at Epes Sargent's suggestion, turned into play form, what had been till then, merely amusing impromptu satires of the peccadilloes of the upper crust's social life, laughingly tossed off for the entertainment of her friends. *Fashion* was written, revised hardly at all, offered to Mr. Simpson of the Park Theatre, accepted, cast, rehearsed, and produced, all within a matter of weeks.

Despite the years of Anna Cora's amateur theatricals, exposure to the real thing was heady stuff and she was instantly entranced.

The procedures for putting a new play into production were dramatically different 140 years ago. Actors read through the play once and then moved about the stage under the direction of the stage manager. Even at the final rehearsal they still clutched their "sides" and were only generally familiar with their lines. Performances resembled a ballet accompanied by the music of words. When an actor entered for the first time, it was almost always on a strong upstage to down, diagonal cross, unless he was very minor indeed, in which case, he might sidle directly on from the wings. Lines were delivered carefully so as to make the most of "points," or the highlights of each speech. The actors who were not speaking froze in suspended animation, whenever someone else was delivering his lines, moving only in between dialogue — no organic, motivational blocking here! Actors were especially careful to avoid turning their backs on their audience. Rehearsal concerns were chiefly taken up with determining the "points" and working out poses in between speeches. The rehearsals usually lasted about a week, during the day. The actors would be performing another play in the evenings. Actors provided most of their own costumes, which were primarily chosen with an eye towards flattery rather than suitability to the role or the period. Scenery usually consisted of a backdrop which represented in a general way, some element of the scene — a garden, a drawing room, etc. — and it was used week after week, whenever an exterior or an interior was called for.[7]

The author was allowed to attend the rehearsals of a new play, but the extensive rewrites common to Broadway tryouts today were unknown. There simply wasn't time. *Fashion* was rehearsed for only a week, and Anna Cora spent most of that time huddled in a darkened box seat off stage wondering what the outcome would be. She was alternately thrilled and appalled. The actors seemed to be working too hard to have the time to indulge in the debauchery with which the theatre was supposed to be rife, and the rehearsal lights shed a dim glow which did not hide the shabby makeshift conditions of even the "Drury Lane of America."

The day of opening dawned. Anna Cora nervously awaited the performance. Rumors about the play had floated in the papers for a week, and all day long, New York's elite had sent for tickets to the play which one of their own had written about THEM! The major critics had all received advance handwritten scripts (which was then the custom) and were to attend. In the house that night, the audience included the mayor, whose house adjoined that of the Mowatts, several other politicians, the Ogden clan, assorted drama critics including Edgar Allan Poe, and "the cream of New York Society, headed by the John Jacob Astors [who] turned out to appraise Mrs. Mowatt's efforts."[8]

Anna Cora was already famous for her brief career as an elocutionist, and for the voluminous literary production of the past years. Her theatrical satire seemed only another step on the path leading straight to notoriety. The *really* big leap was yet to come.

When the curtain rose, Anna Cora crouched in the wings "in case" although what she could do there was unknown. The curtain and the scenery muffled the laughter, and, at first, she was unsure of the play's reception. By the second and third acts, however, it was clear that society had not lost its sense of humor, and by the fifth act curtain, she was already mentally spending her share of the box office receipts.

The critics were ecstatic and vied to outdo each other in praising the play:

> It is with no ordinary feelings of satisfaction that we record the triumphant verdict of the public in favour of Mrs. Mowatt's comedy of *Fashion* ... upon the whole, Mrs. Mowatt may lay claim to having produced the best American comedy in existence, and one that sufficiently indicates her capabilities to write one that shall rank among the first of the age.[9]

> But we hail the production of *Fashion* on higher grounds than mere personal consideration. We believe that the foundation stone is laid by this comedy, for a superstructure that shall prove an enduring monument of the American drama, not merely local in its character, not entirely dependent on home incidents or peculiarities for its construction.[10]

> The unexampled success of this comedy does indeed form an era in the history of the American stage; and we are induced to augur from it the revival of the legitimate Drama. From Mrs. Mowatt we expect much higher achievements than she has exhibited in her first production. She has a loftier mission to fulfill.[11]

Only Edgar Allan Poe expressed reservations about the play:

> [W]e may say that *Fashion* is theatrical but not dramatic. It is a pretty, well-arranged, selection from the usual *routine* of stage characters and stage manoeuvres, but there is not one particle of any nature beyond greenroom nature, about it.... Nor are we quarreling, now, with the more *exaggeration* of character or incident; — were this all, the play, although bad as comedy, might be good as farce, ... Our fault finding is on the score of deficiency of verisimilitude — ...[12]

But after some consideration, he recanted some of his opinions the following week:

> We are delighted to find in the reception of Mrs. Mowatt's comedy, the clearest indications of a revival of the American drama — ... The next step may be the electrification of all mankind by the representation of a *play* that may be neither tragedy, comedy, farce, opera, pantomime, melodrama, or spectacle, as we now comprehend these terms ... it introduces a new class of excellence as yet unnamed because as yet undreamed-of in the world ... this play may usher in a throrough remodification of the theatrical *physique*.[13]

Poe returned to *Fashion* eight times during the next eight performances. His thoughtful analyses of the play are considered to be the true beginnings of the modern art of American dramatic criticism.

Fashion ran for a nearly unprecedented 20 nights at the Park, and Simpson, previously, almost bankrupt, began planning a trip to Europe. James negotiated with a theatre in Philadelphia for *Fashion*'s next production and Anna Cora retired to write another hit.

It wasn't that easy. Day after day passed fruitlessly and Anna Cora succeeded only in ruining her paper and spoiling her pencils. The money from the two successful productions of *Fashion* evaporated, most of it swallowed up in the failure of Mowatt and Co., James' publishing venture. Once again, they were flat broke, and once again, Anna Cora cast about for some new source of income. She was still bedazzled by her recent brush with professional actors and almost impulsively she decided to join their ranks. Instinctively she recognized that she could take advantage of her fame to draw an initial crowd, but that they would have to return because of her skill. She confided her ambitions to Mr. Crisp, who had played in *Fashion*, and he undertook to coach her in the intricacies of the theatre. Together, they chose *The Lady of Lyons* for her debut which was also to be his season benefit. Crisp was no fool. He was relatively unknown, and not yet much of a draw. Adding the notorious Mrs. Mowatt to his cast, in her theatrical bow, virtually guaranteed him a healthy box office.

Anna Cora received most of her preparation from Crisp privately, and had only one rehearsal with the company to prepare her for her first night. She was taking the final step into a profession which no other respectable woman had entered and survived with her reputation unscathed. Anna Cora would change that as well.

[U]nder the stress of necessity, she set about becoming an actress. Friends and relatives protested. For a woman of high social Station to adopt the dubious profession of the stage was little short of a scandal; "but," in her own words, "entreaties, threats, supplicating letters could only occasion me much suffering—they could not shake my resolution."[14]

The Lady of Lyons was a grand melodramtic chestnut, popular throughout the 19th century. Its heroine, Paulina, was ideally suited for Anna Cora's first professional performance, and, despite the recurrence of the nearly paralyzing stage fright which had marked her debut as a "reader," she scored a triumph. If the critics had been pleased by the lady as a dramatist, they were ecstatic with her as an actress: "We have to speak of her acting only in terms of enthusiastic admiration—let her trust proudly to her own grace of manner—her own sense of art—her own rich and natural eloquence."[15] Lawrence Hutton describes the event.

> Her second passage through a "stage door" was when she had her single rehearsal of *The Lady of Lyons* in which she made her debut, and she became an actress and a triumphant one, three weeks after her determination to go upon the stage was formed. Her house was crowded, the applause was genuine and discriminating, and one gentleman, wholly

unprejudiced and of great experience, publicly pronounced it "the best first performance" he ever saw.[16]

It is almost unprecedented for an actress without prior training to make a debut in a leading role in a production mounted in the major theatre of a theatrical center, and to make a resounding success of the effort. "She was one of the few persons of adult years, who going upon the stage without the severe training and long apprenticeship so necessary even to indifferent success, displayed anything like brilliant dramatic qualities. She was an actress and a star born, not made."[17] Only Fanny Kemble was equally unschooled, and *she* was coached for the role of Juliet by Sarah Siddons herself!

Despite her fragile health, Anna Cora was determined to capitalize on her success. James, now acting as her manager, accepted an engagement for her in Philadelphia. Crisp went with her as her leading man. At the Walnut Street Theatre, she repeated *The Lady of Lyons,* played Gertrude in her own *Fashion,* and took roles in several other plays as well. Unfortunately the engagement was not a success. Opening night, Crisp was "unreliable," forgetting lines and wandering about the stage in a peculiar manner, which Anna Cora attributed to stage fright, since she knew he was leery of his reception in the city. The audience was restive and finally began to boo the unfortunate actor. Midway through the play, Anna Cora stepped forward, and out of character, roundly chastised the audience for their unfriendly reception of an out-of-towner. Only after the final curtain fell did another actress tell her that Crisp was drunk! Despite contractual obligations that carried him across America with her for the next nine months, she never spoke to him again.

After Philadelphia, she began a successful series of engagements which carried her to Niblo's Theatre in New York, and to theatres in Buffalo, Boston, and, eventually, to London. Her reputation was growing, and it was constantly enhanced by the critics' praise for her performances. Managers were less interested in the reviews than in the packed houses and overflowing box offices which accompanied Mrs. Mowatt wherever she appeared.

Two novels which she had written previously were brought out by publishers at this time, and sold particularly well, buoyed by her growing fame.

Everywhere she went, she was accompanied by her husband, and since he was devoted to Swedenborgianism,[18] the couple was often seen in church. The more courageous of their friends continued to see the Mowatts, and after some disheartening snubs by acquaintances, she resumed as much of her place in society as her new profession allowed her time for.

Public perception of the character and notoriety of actresses was dealt a severe blow by her continued ladylike demeanor, as Arthur Quinn noted in *A History of American Drama*:

> Real as her contributions to our drama was, her influence upon our theatre was probably even greater. Coming into a life, which notwithstanding the many sterling men and women who pursued it, still suffered from the traditions of loose standards and of the disapproval of the Puritan element in our society, she proved triumphantly that an American gentlewoman could succeed in it without the alteration of her own standard of life. She took into the profession her high heart, her utter refinement, her keen sense of social values and her infinite capacity for effort, and her effect was a real and a great one.[19]

Added Vaughn in *Early American Dramatists*, "she proved that a gentlewoman of taste and breeding could function in the world of the theatre without demeaning herself, thus adding respectability to the profession. And she served notice to the world that America was capable of producing dramatists and actors of consummate skill."[20] "[S]he lived the dubious life of the theatre for nine years without suffering a blemish to her reputation. . . . She had proved that a lady could be an actress and by inference that an actress could be a lady. The status of the profession was materially improved," echoed Hewitt in *Theatre U.S.A.*[21]

A tribute paid her by a group of admirers in Savannah, Georgia, sums up the reactions of the general middle class public: "A lady of your character and attainments elevates and adorns the stage; and we have no doubt that your influence will be widely felt in purifying it from the abuses which sometimes mar its beauties; and that you will cause it to perform its proper task — 'To raise the genius and mend the heart.'"[22] Her biographer Barnes carried matters further with his opinion that

> Being who and what she was, it was inevitable that she should be assigned the mission of making the theatre respectable. If the mission had involved any overt action on her part, she undoubtedly would have shied away from it, for she had none of the impulses of the reformer. But since nothing more was involved than that she be herself, she was willing to let it go at that. She knew that, with a public eager for enjoyment but shackled by a middle-class ideal of respectability, the combination of an impeccable character, recognized social position, and the glamor of the theatre was irresistible.[23]

One of the aspects of her acting which was most commented upon was just that — her acting. In contrast to the recognized "method" of most performers of her time, Mowatt paid less attention to the "points" than to a more naturalistic delivery which required intense study and "character work" to get inside the "skin" of the roles she undertook. She told of coming home from an evening's performance, exhausted and longing to rest, but being forced to study the next day's part to the early hours of the morning, often bathing her temples with ice water or pacing the floor while she studied lines, in order to fully understand and interpret the part she was to play.[24]

> The amount of labor, physical and mental, she endured during this
> period must have been enormous; and the intellectual strain alone was
> enough to have destroyed the strongest mental constitution. *In the history*
> *of the stage in all countries there is no single instance of a mere novice*
> *playing so many important parts so many nights before so many different*
> *audiences, and winning so much and such merited praise,* as did this lady
> during the first twelve months of her career as an actress.[25] (Emphasis
> added.)

The general run of 19th century plays were romantic and melodramatic
and did not as a rule lend themselves much to realistic acting. It would
be a mistake to presume too much upon the comments of the reviewers
of the period. "Naturalistic appearances" notwithstanding, Anna Cora
was not by any means a naturalistic actress in the 20th century meaning of
the words. Although she was not so different as to be obtrusive, we must
still conclude that she was more advanced than many of her fellows.
Moreover she was not adverse to instruction in her craft. In addition to the
lessons from Crisp — including his unintentional one on sobriety and the
stage — she attended elocution lessons in Buffalo — surely unusual in a
"star" — and studiously accepted any criticism offered by the other members
of the company.

She grew very comfortable in performance, the footlights obscuring
the faces of the audience, and during a performance of *School for Scandal*
in New York, even fell asleep on the stage. She was playing Lady Teazle
who first hides behind the screen to avoid discovery by her husband and
then, several pages of dialogue later, is discovered there by Charles Surface. Anna Cora was exhausted by the strenuous string of performances her
success had brought her, and while waiting her cue, stretched out behind
the screen and drifted off. She woke moments later to the frantic calls of
the prompter, scrambled to her feet, and twitched her wig and train into
place seconds before Surface toppled her screen.[26] This may be called the
essence of "ease upon the boards."

Curiously one role she loathed playing was of her own making. Gertrude, the honest but impoverished heroine of *Fashion*, was too insipid for
Anna Cora's chosen type of character, but inevitably she was forced to play
her whenever the play was mounted by a company with which she was
appearing:

> To be forced to enact the walking lady part of Gertrude was a severe
> punishment. To escape its infliction, I always withheld the production of
> the comedy until the solicitations of the public and the managers left me
> no alternative. Could I have foreseen, at the time the play was written,
> that I should be induced to enter the profession, I would have been careful
> to create a character which I could imbody with pleasure.[27]

During her second season in New York, she suffered a freak accident.
Making her exit from a scene, she tripped over a sofa carelessly placed in
the wings. On the arm of the sofa was a pair of hobnailed boots which

caught her in the throat. Nearly collapsing with pain, she made it to her dressing room, completed the costume change, and returned to the stage. Once there, though, all she could do was gasp to E.L. Davenport, her new leading man, "I cannot speak." He went at once to the end of the scene and Anna Cora was helped from the stage, hemorrhaging from a ruptured blood vessel in her throat. Less than two weeks later, still in pain, and only by a superhuman effort of will, she was performing again. There were bills to be paid.

Soon she was also touring again as well—New Orleans, Savannah, Cincinnati, St. Louis and points west. Bates, the owner of the Cincinnati theatre, convinced her to take up her pen again—to write *and* deliver an ode on the opening of his new theatre. The poem celebrated Cincinnati, the theatre, art, poetry, music, and any other suitable sentiments. It was hardly great poetry, but it did stir her long dormant literary urges. She had abandoned writing after her failure to dash off a companion success to *Fashion*. After Cincinnati, she began to write again.

Her motives were personal. After two years of stardom and touring in America, Anna Cora decided that what Charlotte Cushman could do, she could do as well. A London debut was next on her agenda, but she would do Miss Cushman one better. *Her* London bow would be in a play of her own authorship. Accordingly, she created *Armand*, an historical romance which owed little to history and much to romance—19th century style.

It was given a full seven days of rehearsal under Anna Cora's meticulous guidance. As author and star, she now asserted rights she hadn't even known existed two years before during *Fashion's* brief rehearsals. The run of *Armand* at the Park Theatre, despite its success, was really only a dress rehearsal for the *real* opening—in England. It would indeed be seen there, but not for some months.

Anna Cora, James, and E.L. Davenport made a late fall crossing. The weather was unusually rough and the ship was even reported lost. The only engagement James had been able to secure for her was in Manchester. A London manager had offered to see what audiences thought of her and to consider allowing Anna Cora to play in his theatre—"later." The actors of the provincial company were openly hostile to her and the audience absolutely silent during her first performance. Anna Cora was convinced that she had made the major mistake of her career in coming to England. To her surprise, the theatre exploded with applause at the final curtain and the reviews were gracious.

By the time the run in Manchester was finished, the Princess Theatre of London had agreed to admit Davenport and Anna Cora to its company[28] and once more their "crude Americanisms" were to be coldly viewed by hostile British audiences, press and actors. Her debut performance was to be, not *Armand*, which was still being looked at by the Examiner of Plays, but Julia in Sheridan Knowles' *The Hunchback*.

The cast of *The Princess*, with whom she was to play, was even more hostile than the Manchester actors had been, and

> [L]ost no opportunity to tell Mrs. Mowatt how the leading London ac-
> tresses had performed the role of Julia. At one point Anna Cora lost her
> composure and told one of the actors; "Sir, when I have made up my mind
> to become the mere imitator of Mrs. Butler, or of Miss Faucit, or of Mrs.
> Kean, I shall come to you for instruction. At present it is for the public
> to decide upon the faultiness of my conception. . . ."[29]

The actors were undaunted by her feisty response and played cruel tricks on her during performance.

One actor stood with his foot on her train, preventing her from leaping to her feet at one of the dramatic highlights of the play. Also, at the sugges-tion of the management, for her debut she wore a heavily padded corset, designed to give her a more "womanly" figure. Despite these handicaps, the London reviewers were generally kind. "*The Theatrical Times* wrote that she was a 'decided acquisition to the theatre being free from coarseness and Americanisms,'"[30] and as she gave more performances and attracted en-thusiastic crowds, the tenor of the papers became more eulogistic. The main thrust of the praise reveals the general animosity of the British public for American actors. Anna Cora was highly regarded precisely *because* she was so "unlike most Americans" — almost *English* in fact. The reviewers generally corrected her pronunciations of certain words, and she, always eager to learn, obeyed the suggestions until her speech became more like that of those with whom she was appearing.

> Ireland explained her success thus: "Delicacy was her most marked
> characteristic. A subdued earnestness of manner, a soft, musical voice, a
> winning witchery of enunciation, and indeed an almost perfect combina-
> tion of beauty, grace, and refinement fitted her for the very class of
> characters in which Miss Cushman was incapable to excelling, and in
> which *she* commanded the approbation of the British public."[31]

Her understated acting style was not particularly well thought of, but the audiences were able to forgive her, attributing her relatively quiet man-ner in Shakespearian roles to a lack of confidence and training.

As the English embraced Mowatt, she was able to undertake the difficulties of mounting *Armand*. The play was convoluted and im-probable, but full of the bravado and excitement certain to appeal to any audience. And appeal it did. *Armand* has not had the timeless fascination that has kept *Fashion* in production for the last 140 years, but when it opened in London, it was hailed as a masterpiece.

The next year in England mingled triumph and tragedy. Anna Cora starred successfully in a season of productions so highly regarded that she had virtually no female rival on the stage. Personally, however, her life was a shambles. James' old eye disease recurred and he had to be sent to the West Indies to recuperate. While he was there, William Watts, the manager of Anna Cora's theatre, was arrested and jailed for fraud, and his theatres closed. Then Anna Cora suffered a nervous breakdown, or "brain fever." For the next four months she sat in a room reciting nonsense verses or singing off-key.

When she recovered her senses, the horrific events surrounding Watts and his theatres were revealed to her. William Watts was a clerk in an insurance company where his father was a partner. Since youth, he had been fascinated by the theatre and when he saw Anna Cora perform, he was consumed by a drive to be associated with her. To that end, he embezzled money from his business to allow him to lease a theatre, employ a company of actors, create costumes and scenery, and to engage Mrs. Mowatt. At first all went well; the theatre paid its own expenses, and he returned some of the misappropriated funds. If he had not aspired to lavish productions in the newly fashionable, antiquarian style, he might have come out all right, but he "borrowed" and sank ever larger sums into the plays which starred Mowatt. Eventually an audit at his firm revealed his malfeasance. Even so he expected to get off lightly since he was a shareholder in the company and thus, by a technicality in the English law, unable to be charged with theft of money from himself. (That is, his corporation, of which his shares made him part-owner.) The prosecution dodged this loophole with one of its own and charged him with stealing a piece of paper (one that a cheque had been written on, to be sure). He was convicted of that theft and sentenced to ten years' transportation. In a state of shock he returned to his cell and hanged himself. On his nearly naked body, the prison authorities found a miniature of Anna Cora Mowatt and a lock of her hair. The scandal was a wonder in theatrical circles despite Anna Cora's protestations of innocence. Worse was yet to come. Days before he died, James revealed to his wife that he had invested most of her hard-won money in Watts' theatre. It was the third fortune James had lost. The man was not good with money.

James died on February 15, 1851, and was buried near London. Anna Cora was on a provincial tour circuit when word reached her of his death. She resumed playing after the burial and continued until she returned to America. It was James' last wish, expressed in a letter he left for her. Anna Cora did not have good luck with sailing ships either, and like the ship which had brought her to London, the *Pacific* nearly foundered on the voyage home.

Back in New York, she began a series of tours throughout many of the theatrical centers of the country including Boston, New Orleans, Charleston, St. Louis, and Richmond. In Richmond, William Foushee Ritchie, a newspaper editor who had fallen under her spell during an earlier appearance, began romantic pursuit of "the widow Mowatt." At first she was put off by his ardor. Later it came to charm her. On tour, her perennially weak chest began to plague her, and she collapsed with bronchitis. When she recovered, she remembered a promise to James to write her autobiography, and began, feverishly, to do so. It was published in 1854 to nearly universal acclaim. The sole dissenting voice was that of Dr. Mary Walker in *The Evangelical Review*. Despite her advocacy of trousers for women, Dr. Walker was not very advanced in her views. She took exception to Anna Cora's point, in her book, that the theatre and its people were, generally, a very moral, hardworking, and upstanding, group. "How," Dr. Walker asked, "could anyone pretend that the drama was uplifting when, as everyone knows, performances were given at night, and it was at night that passions were susceptible to excitement."[32]

During Anna Cora's farewell tour, her book sold in the theatres and was widely read. She recognized that she no longer had the physical strength to continue on the stage, and in 1854, gave it up after final triumphal appearances on the East Coast. Her last performance was as Paulina in *The Lady of Lyons*. She ended as she had begun.

She also married Ritchie. It was an intimate gathering of just 2,000 invitees, and was "the wedding of the century." When she went to Richmond with her new husband, she found that Southern society was slower than its Yankee neighbors to forgive the taint of the "stage" in a local boy's bride. Once there she divided her time between a new book, *The Mimic Life*, a fictionalized account of life behind the scenes of the theatre, told in three long stories, or novellas, and the campaign to preserve Mount Vernon, the home of George Washington. She allied herself with Ann Pamela Cunningham, the founder of the cause.

Together with other women from Richmond society, they created the Mount Vernon Association, which was chartered by a special act of the Virginia legislature — the first time an association of women was allowed to band together and purchase property, albeit for the benefit of the nation.

Much of the behind-the-scenes politicking for the legislation was done in the Ritchie home and Anna Cora was ecstatic when the bill passed. Now there was only the little matter of raising the $200,000 needed to actually purchase the property. She threw herself into this effort as well, perhaps using it to avoid confronting her husband whom she discovered had made a mistress of one of his family's plantation slaves. Her father was in ill health, nearly 80, and she did not want to break with Ritchie because of the possible effect on him. Samuel Ogden died in April 1860. Shortly after this, while she was still in New York for the funeral, her beloved younger sister Julia fell ill in France, and Anna Cora sailed to take care of her. Julia recovered, but Anna Cora stayed on. When Ritchie came over to retrieve her, she refused to return, precipitating a final break. From Paris she went to Florence, Italy, where she fell in with a band of expatriates of England,

America, and France, and began work on a new novel. Midway through 1862 she returned home. Her money had run out.

She returned to a nation at war. Gallantly, she played the role of a married woman separated from her southern husband by battle lines and loyalties. She did not advertise Ritchie's infidelities and few outside the family circle knew the true state of affairs. She finished *Fairy Fingers*, the novel interrupted by her return to the States, and as her health once more deteriorated, made plans to return to Florence to recover. Before she left, she agreed to become a columnist for papers in Philadelphia, New York, Boston, and Baltimore. Nominally we may, therefore, title her a "foreign correspondent," one of the first women ever to undertake this task. She never returned home.

From Florence she wandered to London, ill, nearly impoverished, and largely forgotten by the cheering crowds of yesteryear. She died at Twickenham on the Thames, near London, on July 27, 1870, and was buried with James at Kensal Green. Almost no one came to the funeral.

Anna Cora Ogden Mowatt Ritchie was a nearly unique figure in the annals of the American theatre. She was a socially prominent figure who defied convention — not once, but repeatedly — to earn a living in the arts and to support her husband. In her own time she was known primarily as a theatrical star, but she is remembered by later generations for two things.

The first, of course, is *Fashion*, that timeless comic classic, as funny in the 20th century as it was in the 19th:

> *Fashion* deserved its success. It is that rare thing, a social satire based on real knowledge of the life it depicts, but painting it without bitterness, without nastiness, and without affectation. It is true to the manners of the time and place, but it is based on human motives and failings that are universal, and when it is placed on the stage today it is as fresh as when it delighted the audiences at the Park Theatre in 1845.[33]

It is the first American play which is interesting and actable in its own right, not merely as an historical curiosity. *Fashion* was very much part of its own time, just as the comedies of Shakespeare were written for a particular cadre of actors, audience and theatre. Both seem ageless to modern audiences. Perhaps their very specificity adds to the universality of the plays.

Secondly, Mrs. Mowatt brought respectability to the stage. She never lost her dignity and she never lost her sense of her place in society and the rights and privileges that were therefore hers. "She was a woman of determination and courage. Her credentials of respectability helped the theatre on its path to acceptance as a tolerable, even honorable profession."[34]

Since she refused to lower herself to fulfill the commonly held opinions of the theatre and actresses, those opinions were, perforce, elevated. We can date the increase in the social acceptance of the actress from the 1840s. No small part of this acceptance is due to Mowatt's influence. It would take another 75 years before the stage became truly respectable, but no longer were critics able to blacken all reputations with a single brush. The stage was very important to Anna Cora Mowatt, and she turned readily to it in times of distress, seeking the fortunes which her talents could provide: "She felt the stage to be her destiny. She determined that her destiny should be fulfilled..."[35] Hutton added, "there flashed across the theatrical sky a meteor of uncommon brilliance ... for nine years [Anna Cora Mowatt] illuminated the dramatic heavens.... Her career ... marks the beginning in the American theatre of the school of emotionalism."[36]

Garff Wilson, in his history of acting in America, sums up Anna Cora Mowatt, the actress and her place in the theatre.

> Mrs. Mowatt was ... a remarkably gifted person. She had unusual intelligence, keen aesthetic perception, thorough education, wide cultural experience, an excellent speaking voice, and beauty of face and figure.... In addition, [she] had an emotional sensitivity which enabled her to "abandon herself to a role...." She wrote, "I never succeeded in stirring the hearts of others unless I was deeply affected myself. The putting off of self-consciousness was, with me, the first important element of success."[37]

Anna Cora Mowatt "was a representative American woman of whom American women have every reason to be proud"[38], "the first American actress to start at the top"[39], "America's first important woman playwright"[40], a "woman of uncommon intelligence and grace, almost a genius"[41], and "a consummate artist"[42]. She was also, of course, a lady.

As Ben Franklin, a crony of her great-grandfather, said:

> If you would not be forgotten
> As soon as you are dead and rotten
> Either write things worth reading
> Or do things worth the writing.

Anna Cora Mowatt did both.

Act II

THE ACTRESSES

In the early decades of theatre in America, few performers enjoyed the luxury of a single occupation. In addition to being an actor, a member of a company turned his hand to everything from carpentry to dancing lessons. During the off-season, he might be a printer or a farmer.

When performances were few or sparsely attended, the local papers would carry announcements by the actors of elocution lessons, fine sewing classes, dancing instructions "including the latest modes," and singing "in the Italian method." When all else failed and revenues were low, the actors were forced the withdraw in a furtive fashion, abandoning props and possessions in a 2:00 A.M. flit which avoided creditors, but did little to enhance the reputation of "the player-folk." When Sol Smith found things in Pittsburgh particularly tough going, he offered each of his creditors a free ticket to the evening's performance, and smuggled the box office take out of the theatre by making a spectacular exit through a trap door in a puff of smoke. He then made his way through the basement of the theatre and to a waiting horse. Presumably the creditors were left to take what pleasure they could from the evening's entertainment. These were the conditions under which Sophia Turner and her companions pursued their art. Their enemies were legion — hostile audiences, hostile conditions, hostile rivals, even hostile Indians! — and their friends few. The playing conditions were crude and the theatres primitive, if they existed at all.

By the time Charlotte Cushman had established herself as the preeminent 19th century American star, these conditions had changed — at least in the major cities — and American theatres could be compared favorably with the finest European houses. Touring was as comfortable as it could be made in those days, and actors in the larger companies rarely had to escape their duns in the dark of night — although they might still be abandoned in midtour by an unscrupulous promoter.

Sophia Turner and Charlotte Cushman were both American leading

37

ladies, and pioneers of the drama. Sophia Turner extended the frontiers of the American theatre while Charlotte Cushman conquered the challenges posed by English snobbery. The one broadened the scope of the theatre within the growing borders of the United States, the other helped the theatre achieve maturity and respect outside those borders.

The extent to which conditions had changed in a relatively short time (less than 40 years) owes more to the hardihood of the performers than to any external reforms. Were it not for these stalwart souls, the westward expansion of the country would have been a much drearier and less appealing prospect. Hard, exhausting, backbreaking, unremitting labor was all that enabled the pioneers to wrest New Orleans, Mobile, Albany, Cleveland, and the multitude of towns in between, from the vast forests and uncrossable rivers. Touring companies of actors — whether performing scapegrace comedies, or high tragedies, whether on stages in taverns, or in elegantly appointed theatres — leavened the toil with laughter and drama, and played their part in the growth of the nation.

Sophia Turner

Pittsburgh had a severe shortage of virgins. That's what a theatrical company playing there in 1815 discovered when they presented *Pizarro*, an earlier version of *Royal Hunt of the Sun*, which required a large number of vestal virgins for a scene. The citizens of that brawling river town would sooner have floated down the Ohio in a barrel than set foot on the stage. Eventually the cast was fleshed out by the addition of the washer-woman who cleaned the theatre and the stage carpenter, both tastefully draped in cheesecloth.

"Oh, what *virgins!*" an irrespressible sailor exclaimed from the pit and pandemonium ensued.[1]

Bizarre as this episode may seem in comparison to modern theatrical practices, it was typical of the early itinerant troupes pushing westward with a handful of scripts, a few rags of costumes, and an overwhelming determination to carry their performances to an entertainment-starved people.

They followed virtually in the footsteps of the pioneers, and by the first decade of the 1800s, theatres flourished, albeit often briefly, in the burgeoning riverfront towns whose establishment were signposts in the westward growth of America. Pittsburgh, Cincinnati, and St. Louis all proudly acknowledged "theatrical palaces" dedicated to entertaining their folk. Interestingly, each of these mercantile and artistic centers had their first encounters with professional theatre with the same company of actors — a company whose leading lady was Sophia Turner. As word of their success filtered back to the playhouses in New York and Philadelphia, other actors followed Sophia, eager to emulate her triumphs. The company was under the management of Sophia's husband, William A. Turner, who also performed when necessary.

William and Sophia crossed the Atlantic from England and then, after a brief season in New York, pushed steadily west—Montreal to St. Louis and countless hundreds of settlements and army outposts and taverns in between. Everywhere they went, they carried their profession with them, playing for a few coppers, a meal, a place to sleep.

They must often have been exhausted, hungry and frightened. They traveled a thousand miles and more over impossible and frequently impassable roads. "There was no way for theatrical companies from the East to reach Pittsburg [sic] prior to 1817, save by the state road which was scarcely passable for a train of pack horses, yet they came as early as 1803 and performed in a small room which was secured for them when the court room was occupied."[2] They wheedled passage from unenthusiastic riverboat captains and slept, sometimes five to a bed, in the redlight districts. Wherever America's pioneers had established settlements, they were followed by actors eager to relieve the danger and the tedium of building a nation. The first of these groundbreaking companies was the one established by William Turner, starring his wife Sophia. For a few brief years, Sophia Turner was *the* leading lady west of the Alleghenies.

When Sophia Turner was playing the riverfront towns of the West, there was a recurring similarity to the company's activities. Once in a town large enough to ensure an audience, William Turner, as manager, would secure a performance space, sometimes a large meeting room, or a barn, or an outdoor market area where a stage could be contrived. The actors would personally distribute the handbills and broadsides, nailing them up wherever there was a vacant tree. Rehearsals would be held in the makeshift "theatre" and when an audience had congregated and the price of admission had been extracted from them, the performance would begin.

Customarily there was a large dramatic piece, followed by a farce with musical and dancing interludes throughout. Performances began around 6:30 P.M. and ended many hours later. The players would stay in a town so long as there was a paying audience for their wares, and then it was off to the next village with its barn or meeting hall.

Wherever she appeared, the newspapers carried testimonials to the talent of the leading lady and polish of her performance. An early "critic" praised her. "[She has] a truly beautiful face and elegant figure (forming together a graceful and expressive contour)—the tear glistening eyes, the repeated plaudits of the audience evince the excellence of her acting."[3] The few appraisals of the competence of the actors who supported her which survive are "mixed," but the praise for her performances was universal:

> Mrs. Turner possesses considerable talents and powers, with grace, ease
> and elegance combined, and a person beautiful and fascinating; an au-
> dience of taste can but be interested in whatever part she may under-
> take. . . . [T]he buffoonery and babboon [sic] capers of some of the others
> have been ill timed, but will do well in their proper place.[4]

Sophia Turner was born in England, sometime before 1785 to 1790,
and played at the Drury Lane, London and the Theatres Royal, Bath and
Bristol[5], before she and her husband, William, who does not seem to have
originally been an actor, left for New York. She appeared at the Park
Theatre, New York, in a "brief, inconsipicuous career on these classic
boards"[6] in the role of Angela in The Castle Spectre in September 1807. In
1808 she played Miranda in William Dunlap's production of The Tempest.[7]
This may have been the highlight of her first appearance at the Park.

After the season in New York, she and William moved to The Theatre,
managed by John Mills, in Montreal. There they performed with Mr. Kennedy and Mr. and Mrs. Cipriani who would form the nucleus of the fledgling Turner company. On July 16 they appeared in a performance of Lover's
Vows by Mrs. Inchbald, with David Douglas,[8] and three days later Mrs.
Turner was given a benefit of Laugh When You Can with the farce The
Spoiled Child. As always Sophia was well thought of — "Sophia Turner was
ladylike in her deportment on the stage and showed great professional
culture,"[9] but William failed to impress anyone ("his individual merit was
said to be in cooking canvas-back ducks").[10] Small wonder that William left
the stage to his more talented wife whenever possible.

From Montreal, the majority of the company headed south, arriving
in Lexington, Kentucky, by December 15, 1810. It is possible that they went
by way of Philadelphia since Brown in his History places Sophia on the
stage there in October of 1810.[11] Lexington was one of the oldest towns on
the frontier. When the actors from "Montreal and Quebec" arrived to perform, their audience probably included students from Transylvania College, the oldest educational institution west of the Alleghenies. The town
was the center of a growing tobacco industry, and had been a territorial
capital. This mix of government, business, and education provided a fertile
audience for the theatre. No wonder there was so much dispute over the
Kentucky circuit. The climate was excellent, the audiences supportive, and
the habit of play-going well established.

The actors advertised themselves as "a company of theatrical performers from Montreal and Quebec"[12] and were under the nominal
management of James Douglas. The "theatrical performers" included the
Turners, the Ciprianis, and Kennedy and Douglas from Montreal together
with some other actors they acquired en route.[13]

The company played in Lexington about two weeks and then on
Christmas Day they journeyed to Frankfort, Kentucky, where they stayed

for the better part of a month. Frankfurt was established on the river in 1786 by a handful of settlers. The capital of the territory, and, later, the state, it was located in the rolling bluegrass hills, and its residents thought it the pleasantest spot on earth. After the hellish journey from the frozen wilds of Canada, the Turners probably agreed with them. The company ran through their repertory for the citizens of Frankfurt, playing once or twice a week. Their performances were well enough attended to keep them in town for over four weeks, but, by the end of January 1811, they had decided to return to Lexington.

The theatre they established in Lexington lasted until spring. The actors performed for the next three months until there was a disagreement which caused the breakup of the company. The Turners and the Ciprianis announced publicly that they would no longer be associated with the other players.[14] This may have been an early publicity stunt, however, because within a week they were performing *Othello* and a farce with the full cast. When the season ended, though, the Turners and Ciprianis went on to Cincinnati and did not rejoin their colleagues for the short summer season in Lexington. Evidently Sophia's talents as a leading lady were sorely missed because the company had to round out their casts with amateurs in the women's roles, despite the addition of "Mrs. Jordy" to the roster.[15]

"Certainly the outstanding talent in Lexington's first professional season was Mrs. Sophia Turner, who drew exceptionally favorable notices for her roles. She was undoubtedly the first actress of real merit to visit the West."[16]

Cincinnati, the "Queen City," wasn't even a city when Sophia Turner first appeared on the stage there. The settlement was less than 30 years old, and its residents were far more interested in the price of hogs than in theatrical bills. Wherever the Turners went, the streets of London receded further behind them. The metropolitan delights of England must have seemed very far away indeed in a village whose pedestrians had to fight for walking space with hogs on their way to market. Cincinnati was the greatest hog market in the country and the streets were filled with pigs driven on foot from Ohio and Indiana to the slaughterhouses which were responsible for the stench which always hung over the town. Cincinnati was on the river, and its main business was shipping pork back to Philadelphia and New York. The influx of "ham" from the theatres of the East, was a welcome change.

In Cincinnati, William Turner began his career as a manager. He presented several performances during May and June of 1811. The company starred Sophia and included the Turner children and the Ciprianis whose specialty was dancing, and who offered dancing lessons wherever they were appearing.

They established their theatre "near the Columbian Inn" and began their brief season near the end of May with a performance of *Animal Magnetism* by Mrs. Inchbald. The farce which followed was Colman's *The Wag of Windsor*. In addition to the two plays, there were songs, dances, hornpipes, and a recitation by Mrs. Turner. It was a lot of entertainment for seventy-five cents. Evidently the offering was so popular that tickets were oversold and not all those who held tickets were able to see the performance, since several days later, the company printed an announcement guaranteeing "that efficient means are being taken to prevent any further disturbances." A few days later, the company played *Douglas* and *The Romp*. Sophia Turner starred as Lady Randolph, but a nameless amateur was recruited from Lexington for Young Norval. In fact William was desperately short of professional actors and had to resort repeatedly to amateurs with doubtful expertise. He had "several gentlemen of Cincinnati" in the cast of *Secrets Worth Knowing* and another "Cincinnati gentleman" as the lead, Mungo, in *The Padlock*, which with revival of *Douglas* concluded his first Cincinnati season. Although he had the talents of the Ciprianis, and his own children, only Sophia was a skilled actress and performer.[17] This original group was ill-assorted, lacked leading men and character women, and needed fleshing out generally if it was to present the kinds of plays which would appeal to the audiences of the frontier towns. William and Sophia quickly recognized this and changed their strategy accordingly. They decided to return East, regroup, and add to the company.

Although the first foray into Cincinnati was not sufficient to maintain the company there for long, they would return periodically until the final battle with Sam Drake over the territory. The actors performed briefly in Lexington on their way to Pittsburgh where they announced performances during the fall.

They remained there throughout the winter months, performing at weekly intervals. William Turner induced some of the wealthier townspeople to join him in creating a building devoted to theatre[18] and a subscription base was established. Professional theatre had come to Pittsburgh.

Pittsburgh was not yet the sprawling medical-mining-industrial complex it would become. In 1812, it was still primarily what it had been established as, when George Washington surveyed it in 1753 — the fortified garrison at the confluence of three rivers; the gateway to the West; and the trading post at the end of civilization.

Because of the location's mercantile importance, wealth and population were already starting to concentrate in the settlement around Fort Pitt. In 1812, however, a second war with the British had broken out and Pittsburghers followed it closely. The weekly papers printed verbatim dispatches from the conflict and the community was on the alert for a British fleet sailing down the Monongahela.

Small wonder they gave little attention to the theatrical delights advertised by William Turner which were sandwiched in among notices of potash sales, $10 rewards for runaway horses and six-cent rewards for runaway mulattoes, on the back pages of *The Mercury*.

Nevertheless, William succeeded in raising interest and capital and in May 1812, he advised, in the *Gazette*, that subscriptions were to be paid in thirds — one-third on May 8, one-third on May 25, and one-third on June 8.[19]

By November 1813, however, William was advertising "To be sold: One Moiety or ½ part of the Pittsburgh Theatre with scenic decorations, embellishments, etc. From the receipts of the theatre it holds out a very valuable prospect to a purchaser. A considerable deduction will be made in the consideration money for cash."[20] Whether this was the Turners' share of the theatre, or simply an attempt to raise more cash for productions is not clear.

During their seasons in Pittsburgh, the company performed an extraordinarily broad range of material which testifies both to Sophia's versatility as an actress and to the ambition of a company which permitted neither lack of personnel nor lack of suitability to prevent them from tackling the kinds of plays popular in London and New York. At least at first, their audiences were enthralled.

Almost none of the standards of their repertory would be recognizable to a modern audience, but they were performed by virtually every troupe of actors in the late 18th and early 19th centuries. On September 23, 1813, the company opened with *The Monk*, a gothic tragedy liberally sprinkled with spectral figures, a complex plot, horrible occurrences, and general mayhem, by Matthew Gregory "Mad Monk" Lewis. If Stephen King and Steven Spielberg were ever to collaborate on a stage piece, the result might be something very like *The Monk*. Once the audiences were thoroughly terrorized, they were then treated to *The Weathercock*, a farce. Always leave 'em laughing.

The next week, Sophia Turner and the others wowed the audience with *Pizarro* (or) *The Death of Rolla*, a grand old melodramatic tragedy by Kotzebue, translated and adapted by Richard Brinsley Sheridan. *Pizarro* was one of the warhorses of the early American theatre, played over and over again, in every imaginable playhouse, under every imaginable condition from the Park Theatre in New York, to a crude barn somewhere in the Midwest. It called for spectacular scenic effects, and of course, *those* virgins, and the Pittsburgh Theatre was not above letting their audiences know what to expect.

The following extract of the plot is taken verbatim from their advertisement in the *Mercury* on September 30, 1813. Mrs. Turner took the part of Cora.

Act One, Scene First — A magnificent pavilion near Pizarro's tent, with a view of the Spanish camp in the background. Elvira discovered sleeping.

Act Two, Scene First A grove. Cora discovered playing with her child.

Scene 2d The Temple of the Sun, representing Peruvian idolatry — in the center is the altar — A solemn march. The warriors and King enter on one side of the Temple — Rolla, Alonzo and Cora on the other — A Ball of Fire descends upon the altar — The whole ensemble rise and join Thanksgiving.

Act III — Scene 1st A wild retreat amongst the rocks — Cora and her child discovered — A triumphant march of the army is heard at a distance. The King, Rolla and soliders enter — Cora with her child in her arms runs through the ranks searching and inquiring for Alonzo

3d — Pizarro's tent. Pizarro discovered traversing the scene in gloomy and ferocious agitation.

Act IV Scene 1st — A dungeon in the rock near the Spanish camp. Alonzo in chains — a centinel [sic] walking near the entrance — Rolla enters in disguise and implores Alonzo to exchange his dress: who after much entreaty puts on Rolla's disguise, passes the centinel, [sic] and escapes.

Act V — 1st — A thick forest. In the background a hut almost covered with boughs — A dreadful storm, with thunder and lightning. Cora had covered her child in a bed of leaves — her appearance is wild and distracted. While she is wrapping her veil over him, Alonzo's voice is heard at a distance — Cora anxiously looking for his approach — Two Spanish soldiers enter and carry away the child. She returns with Alonzo and runs to the spot where she had left the child: but finding it gone, she shrieks and stands in speechless agony.

Scene 2d The subposts of the Spanish camp — the background wild and rocky with a torrent falling down a precipice, over which a bridge is formed by a fallen tree. Rolla in chains is brought in by the soldiers — other soldiers bring in the child which Rolla, perceiving it to be Cora's, supplicates Pizarro to save and protect it. Pizarro refusing, Rolla seizes the child, and crosses the bridge, pursued by Spanish soldiers — they fire at him — a shot strikes him — Pizarro exclaims "Now! quick! quick! seize the child!" Rolla tears from the rock the stone that supports the bridge and retreats, wounded, bearing off the child in triumph to Ataliba's tent, where, bleeding, he enters pursued by Spanish soldiers — delivers the child to Cora and expires —

After which a much admired farce, called
Of Age To-Morrow[21]

Whatever the Pittsburgh Theatre's presumption of the unsophistication of their audiences, such an advertisement of the spectacles and wonders to be performed must have taken some living up to.

This performance was followed a week later by a comic opera, *The Highland Reel,* and on October 14, 1813, Mrs. Turner played Juliet to Mr. Kennedy's Romeo. Two months later, she starred as Belvidera in *Venice Preserv'd.*

There are no formal reviews extant of the company during their time in Pittsburgh. Nevertheless, there are a number of assumptions which may be made about this professional troupe of actors during this time. First of all, they played material which appealed to their audiences, mingling classics like *Romeo and Juliet* and *Venice Preserv'd* with popular "modern" works like *Pizarro* and *The Spoiled Child.*

Secondly, the actors were truly versatile. For example, Sophia Turner alternated between a role in a gothic masterpiece like *The Monk* and *singing* the lead in *The Highland Reel.* One week she was lovelorn, teenaged Juliet, the next, a distracted, motherly Cora. The other actors were equally at home in farce, tragedy, melodrama, and comic opera. This argues for great skill on their part, or great tolerance from the audience.

Thirdly, all of their plays called for large casts and even if their company doubled and tripled the roles, they must have been forced to use whoever in the community was willing to risk their reputations with "the players." Probably these performers were drawn from members of the two amateur dramatic societies. Evidently actors were interchangeable between the amateurs and the professionals. For example, Mrs. Barrett appeared with both the Turners and the amateur thespians in the same year.[22]

Finally, the most difficult aspect of the productions must have been the scenery. Such marvels as were promised in *Pizarro* could not have been easy to come by for the company. The addition of John Vos (or Voss) in Cincinnati at least added a scene painter to the group but until then William and Sophia probably devised their own. To provide the kind of spectacular delights which were promised, must have strained the resources of the company to the utmost. Perhaps the outlay required was the beginning of the end for the Turners. Less than six weeks later William was seeking to raise cash. Even as poorly conceived as the effects must have been that the Turners could create, they whetted the appetite of the audiences for the more spectacular effects and newer plays which the companies which followed them could provide. In their turn, these companies were supplanted by larger, more elaborate groups as the sophistication of the theatres, the audiences, and the troupes grew. Eventually the older, and less well-equipped companies simply stopped being able to compete.

The theatre buildings were part of this trend. William Turner created the idea of having a group of businessmen subscribe to build a theatre, and this idea was elaborated on across the frontier. In some locations, the theatres in which these pioneering acting companies performed were as rickety and gim-cracked as the wobbly scenery. In others, they were quite spectacular. No descriptions still exist of Pittsburgh's first theatre, or indeed of the first theatres of most of the frontier towns, but they were for the most part, small structures capable of being adapted to many uses.

The players remained in Pittsburgh at least until the end of 1813, and when Turner took his company on the road again, they were known as "The Pittsburgh Company of Comedians," a title he retained despite residencies in several other towns. He was justly proud of the company he had engaged. Although some were relative unknowns, several were popular favorites from eastern stages. Mrs. George Barrett was a well-known English character actress who had begun her career as a protégé of Charles Macklin, and performed in New York theatres since 1798. Another recruit was Thomas Jefferson, son of Joseph Jefferson, one of the earliest leading men of the American stage, and grandfather of Joseph Jefferson who became renowned for his roles as Rip Van Winkle, and Asa Trenchard in *Our American Cousin* (see pg. 79–80), and who ended his career touring with Mrs. John Drew in *The Rivals* (see p. 100).

Thomas Caulfield was another English actor whose services Turner succeeded in engaging. Caulfield had performed at the Drury Lane and the Park Theatre, and was known as a mimic and a hypochondriac. However, one of his "imaginary illnesses" caught up with him, and he died in Cincinnati while performing with the Turners. Joshua Collins, who began his career with William and Sophia, was a talented actor who overcame his unprepossessing physique to play most of Shakepeare's tragic heroes. Collins went on to play with Drake and to manage theatres in many Midwestern towns. Turner also added several couples, the Milners and Morgans, and a number of "utility gentlemen" to his company.[23]

When the Pittsburgh Company of Comedians was at full strength, Turner carried out his promise to the people of the frontier towns to recruit "performers of the first celebrity on the continent, in addition to those whose talents are now offered to their attention."[24] As T. Hill West notes, "this statement . . . was in some measure carried out by Turner, who managed to recruit at least two foreign stars and several excellent supporting players for his company."[25]

By 1814, they were back in Lexington where Turner assumed the management of the remnants of the company abandoned there several years before. He added them to his newly recruited actors and played a circuit of theatres in Lexington, Frankfurt, and Louisville.[26] The following year, he enlarged the circuit to include Cincinnati, and the Turners enjoyed the greatest relative prosperity they had had since coming to America. It didn't last.

> William Turner had managed to organize the largest and most talented theatrical group ever witnessed by western audiences. Not only did he have a reserve of supporting actors, but he had a substantial variety of leading players, including Mrs. Turner, Mrs. Barrett [and] Collins. . .[27]

However, their time in Lexington ended bitterly when Turner was forced to yield his theatre because of the duplicity of Luke Usher who had made virtually simultaneous rental agreements with William Turner and Sam Drake. The Turners' bitterness was evident when they advertised "positively the very last night . . . by the present company, and Mrs. Turner's last appearance in Lexington." The Turners were leaving Kentucky behind.[28]

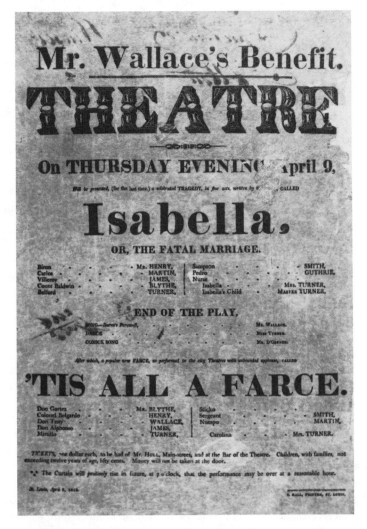

Playbill for the production of "Isabella" at Wallace's Theatre, April 9, 1818 (courtesy of the Missouri Historical Society).

Sam Drake and Noah Ludlow were among those who had been eyeing the success of the "Pittsburgh Company of Comedians," and they began their career by following in the footsteps of the earlier actors. Their company was larger, better-equipped, and, most important of all to the audiences, unfamiliar. They began by invading Pittsburgh before the Turners returned to Kentucky. Drake followed, and Turner retreated to Cincinnati when he was forced to abandon the other lucrative playhouses in Kentucky. Drake and Ludlow, in the pattern they would follow across the Midwest, invaded a city, produced the same plays, hired away the most promising of the actors and took over the audiences which had been carefully built by Sophia Turner's fine performances.

Ludlow, in his autobiography, admittedly written many years later, did not hesitate to denigrate the company he was supplanting.

> We found in Cincinnati a small company under the management of Mr. Turner . . . but owing to a long term of bad business he had not been able to pay the salaries of his actors and consequently there was nothing but complaint and insubordination among them. . . . When Mrs. Turner's benefit came on the house was full, and it was said that many paid for tickets who could not get in the small ill-contrived place they called a theatre. This building, erected for some other purpose than a theatre . . . was approached by a long flight of rough plank steps, up which an audience had to ascend and descend at the imminent peril of their limbs and life. . . . Mr. Turner was not an actor.[29]

Much of the credit for carrying theatre west is often given to Ludlow, Sol Smith, and Sam Drake, and they do deserve praise, but the attention directed toward their companies has largely obscured the very real contributions of those who preceded them. When examining the history of the early territorial theatres, similar occurrences are evident. William and Sophia Turner and their children, together with a few half-trained actors, would establish an audience and a theatre space. As their success increased, other theatrical troupes would appear to vie for business. Not surprisingly, the audiences would be attracted to the company whom they had not seen and who advertised themselves as having the "newest plays." In short order, the Turners would have to move on again. At least once, Drake bought the lease of a theatre which had already been promised to William Turner, and Turner took the matter to court.[30] Of course, it didn't matter. In the interim, the Turners and the remaining members of the Pittsburgh Company of Comedians had already been driven out of town and their best actors incorporated into the Drake Ensemble.

Stubbornly Turner hung on in Cincinnati until the end of 1817, and then, with Drake snapping at his heels, left for St. Louis where he converted a building which had variously been a blacksmith shop and then a courthouse and even a church, into "The Theatre."[31] He incorporated the stable loft of a nearby tavern into the performance space (perhaps as a balcony), and opened a season there which ran through the spring and summer months.

St. Louis had only been a part of the United States for a short period of time. In 1804 it was added to the territories as a piece of the Louisiana Purchase, and its streets were still crowded with a multinational cadre of fur traders, keelboaters, and explorers. The biggest business in town was the American Fur Company and the Missouri River was the main "highway." The fixed population was small and many of those attending

"The Theatre" to cheer Turner's performances were having a final fling before they began the greatest series of explorations in the history of man.

The audiences were largely composed of men dressed in buckskins, smelling of the bears they'd recently killed, and women who had lost most of their respectability somewhere east of Illinois, and who were nearly as gamey and hard-bitten as their men. Actors who played this town were exposed to audiences whose likes had never been seen in the East. These were men and women who lived hard, fought fair, played rough, and died young, and they expected the plays they saw to be at least as exciting as their own lives. It was the toughest of all possible audiences.

The St. Louis Theatre was a kind of last hurrah for William and Sophia Turner. They performed the tragedy *Bertram* on February 17, 1818, for their opening, and followed it up with other performances at irregular intervals including *Isabella* for the benefit of Mrs. Turner. Their company included at least 16 actors, although some of them may have been local amateurs recruited in St. Louis. Mr. Vos was still with the Turners, but the Ciprianis had defected.[32]

As always, the chief attraction of the Turner company was the talented leading lady. The *Missouri Gazette* of February 20, 1818, carried the following glowing description of her performance.

> Mrs. Turner's Imogine.... The more I see of this ladies [*sic*] acting, the more I am pleased with it. With all the advantages of a personal beauty and a finished education, her long experience enables her to fill with credit every department of the drama, and to feel at home in whatever she performs. Her Imogine presented a lively picture of a chaste and honorable woman, whose excessive sensibility and high-wrought enthusiasm, drives her down the rough tide of calamity, till she is dashed to pieces on the rock of her own distempered feelings. The passions that tortured the heart of Imogine are such that no woman can endure and live. The progress of her sufferings from grief to despair, from despair to frenzy, and from frenzy to death, was sketched with a boldness of coloring, and a felicity of execution which evinced Mrs. T's deep knowledge of the human heart, and her admirable skill in controlling pulsations.[33]

No wonder, years later "A Friend of the Drama" cautioned the residents of St. Louis about Ludlow's troupe:

> We must not look for performers here to equal those in the Atlantic cities; neither must we expect to find a Mrs. Turner. Mrs. T. had not her superior as an actress in the United States...[34]

The season was not profitable, and finally William and Sophia acknowledged defeat and returned to the East where Sophia appeared on the New York stage once more. There was a roughly seven-year gap between Mrs. Turner's last recorded appearance in St. Louis, and November 1825 when she joined the company of Lafayette's Amphitheatre in New York. She spent part of that time playing her way back east, by way of New Orleans where her husband had spoken of opening a theatre.

T. Hill West, in his book *The Theatre in Early Kentucky*, says "In March 1819 the Turners were acting in New Orleans after having performed in almost every community west of the Allegheny Mountains."[35]

In 1826, Sophia joined Edwin Forrest, Charles Durang, and Mary Ann Duff at the Bowery Theatre. It was a company the *Mirror* called "the best in the country."[36] Certainly the theatre was among the most advanced. It was lit with gas jets, housed in ground glass, then a most modern invention. However, Mrs. Turner seemed to be on a downward spiral in her career. The Lafayette, and the Bowery, were not in the same class as the Park Theatre where she'd played in 1807, and the same 1826–27 season found her appearing with an equestrian troupe both at the Bowery and at Lafayette's.

During the summer in 1827 she appeared at the Chatham Garden which closed the following March. Here she seems to have played first and second roles, albeit at a third rate theatre — the Widow in *The Road to Ruin*, Lady Duberly in *The Heir at Law*, and one of the Pickles in *The Spoiled Child*, with Miss Riddle as Little Pickle. The Chatham was a minor theatre and evidently it was a struggle to make a living while in its employ, for on December 26, 1827,

> Mrs. Turner . . . promised at the corner of Reed St. (Boisseux's Dancing Academy, Reed St. and Broadway) a series of amateur concerts which she grandly styled "Convito Armonico." On January 14th . . . she regrets that severe illness in her family forced her to postpone her concert to January 23rd . . . [she advertised] her "Evenings at Home" readings (chiefly from Scott's longer poems) for "twelve nights" at 51 Canal St., the first date of advertising being Feb. 11th. She endured at least till April 9th, when the Post of the 10th advertises her "Convito Armonica" at 440, Corner, Broome and Broadway — the third site, thus far of her moving temple of art.[37]

The Chatham Garden had been closed for two months when Maywood took over the management on June 9, 1828, and opened the season with *The Rivals*. Sophia Turner played Mrs. Malaprop and "the company was undoubtedly the best of the three so far associated with the house during the present season — perhaps the best since that famous one of the summer and autumn of 1824. Its excellence is shown with its opening bill of June 9th . . ."[38] Whatever Maynard's intentions, by July 30 the company was reduced to performing novelty acts like *Monster and Magician*. It was back to the circus again and a sorry comedown for a woman who had once been the toast of the West. On August 1, the Chatham company failed and (presumably) Mrs. Turner left the stage for good.[39] In 1830 William Turner entered the printing business in Philadelphia with his son Frederick. The Turners were now abandoning the stage which had already abandoned them. Sophia Turner died outside Philadelphia in 1852 or 1853. By then she would hardly have recognized the towns she had barnstormed through 40 years before.

Sophia Turner's origins are obscure. She was the wife of William Turner, a sometime printer, actor, and manager. She had three children, a daughter Emma, and two sons, William and Frederick. She taught elocution and acted in third rate roles in New York, and she died near Philadelphia after 1852. In sum this is the total of her life and were it not for those tumultuous years opening theatres wherever dreams of land and glory had taken the brawling, adventurous citizens of America, she would have vanished utterly like Miss Dellinger, Mr. Bancker, and Mrs. Kenna, who do not even rate footnote citation in the most detailed history of the American theatre.

Whatever the shortcomings of her company, it was immensely popular wherever it performed. Much of this popularity may be attributed to the charm and talents of its leading lady: "words seemed to flow from the impulses of feeling rather than from memory. In short her genius for the stage seems general and good in both comedy and tragedy. Her pronunciation and delivery are just and clear, her cadence musical..."[40]

Here we have Sophia Turner, a woman and an actress. It took particular courage and devotion to the theatre to spend years in the worst conditions, without a permanent home, shooting game from dressing room windows for dinner, raising children in the backstage, and living out of trunks, and for what? The chance to perform an all-too-familiar role for the thousandth time, on a makeshift stage with a company composed partly of amateurs, for an audience which, while appreciative, did not have any *real* understanding of the artistry and rigors involved in the production. Sophia Turner was consumed by the magic of the stage, and across the frontier, there were countless thousands of people who shared just a little of that magic as they watched her perform. For just a few hours they were transported to another realm, another world, another life. That was the art of Sophia Turner, the First Actress of the Frontier.

Charlotte Cushman

"She was considerable of a woman, for a play-actress"[1]

Mount Auburn Cemetery lies slightly north of Boston, overlooking the Charles River. It is a lonely place, as most graveyards are, full of ghostly memories and forgotten people. There is a faint breeze. On the rise a cold, white, marble obelisk faces the city. There are no dates carved into it, no touching sentiments. The monument bears only two words— a name. It was a name expected to echo down the centuries, to resound in theatre lobbies across the land, to be whispered whenever the curtain rose on an evening's entertainment. More than a century has passed. Fame's

fleeting touch is no more. All is quiet in this forlorn place. All is forgotten.

Consider, if you will, this scenario for a prototypical Horatio Alger
story: "A poor, but talented, young person of aristocratic lineage, seeks to
earn an honest living upon the stage. At first the obstacles appear insur-
mountable — lack of training, parental disapproval, even vocal failure, but,
one by one, she conquers them, until, at last, she stands on the pinnacle
of success, renowned by all, admired by her fellows, and lauded by the
critics. She dies rich, beloved, and famous."

Incredibly this is one story Alger didn't have to invent. Charlotte
Cushman really did drag victory from the clutches of defeat, and buoyed
only by her unconquerable faith in herself, became an international star,
as sought after in England and Rome as in her native America.

How is it possible that a woman who was notoriously plain in an era
when a pretty face was the *least* requirement for a stage career, whose
voice, while tremendously versatile, was often called hollow and sepulchral,
and who was tall, broad-shouldered and commanding, in a generation of
play-actresses who simpered, fluttered and fainted, was able to dominate
the stages of New York and London to universal acclaim?[2]

Quite simply Charlotte Cushman was too far from the mainstream in
appearance and demeanor to settle comfortably into a niche as a utility
player/leading lady. "Great Success' or "Complete Failure" were the only
routes open to someone as original as she. Failure was personally unaccept-
able so she bent her considerable talents and all her remarkable energies
toward success. Inevitably success succumbed, swooning neatly at her feet
in the person of dozens of fawning critics who could find no fault with Miss
Cushman as Lady Macbeth, as Meg Merrilies, as Nancy Sykes, as Queen
Katharine, as Romeo, as Hamlet . . .

Charlotte accepted this adulation as her just due, owed her by virtue
of her struggles and her talents. Worship was only appropriate: "I like
William [Winter, a major 19th century critic] because he puts me *up* where
I belong."[3]

It all began humbly enough in 1790 when Erasmus Babbitt, a fiddle-
playing Yankee lawyer who always preferred music to mortgage liens and
who was ever ready to play a tune, but reluctant to try a court case, married Mary Saunders of Gloucester. Her family was connected with the Win-
throps, the Sergeants and the Saltonstalls. The match produced three
children. Erasmus gave his children and grandchildren his talent, but
couldn't seem to manage to feed them very often. In 1810, his wife, fed up
with his vagaries, moved to Boston where she opened a boarding house and
her daughter, Mary Eliza, gave music lessons.[4]

A prosperous, middle-aged merchant must have seemed the answer to
their prayers. Mary Eliza wasted no time marrying Elkanah Cushman,

widower, father of two grown children, and descendant of a Mayflower voyager. Their first child, Charlotte, was born the following July 23, 1816. The Cushman name was a well-known one in New England in the early years of the 19th century.

The family began in America when Robert Cushman arrived in the New World in 1621 on board the *Fortune,* second ship to dock in Plymouth Bay. In short order he preached the first sermon heard in the Massachusetts colony and his son Thomas married Mary Allerton from the *Mayflower.*[5]

By the sixth generation, the blood had thinned a little along with the family fortunes. Although some branches had prospered, Elkanah's wasn't one of them, and he found himself an orphan on a hardscrabble farm, penniless and alone.[6] He hiked to Boston, found employment and settled into working his way toward owning a thriving shipping firm. This early effort had an adverse effect on his later years. Mary Eliza wasn't to know this until it was too late, and the prospect of marrying into New England aristocracy (the *Mayflower* descendants) and taking the place in society to which her blood entitled her and which had been denied her by her father's tuneful indolence, warmed Mary Eliza's social-climbing heart as much as the heaviness of Elkanah's purse.

Scarcely had she presented him with the first of five offspring than she was forced to acknowledge some hard truths. Elkanah Cushman, far from being the moneyed, hard-working businessman she thought she'd snared, was turning out to be another wastrel like her father. Grimly, she and her mother set out to salvage what they could from the wreckage of his business, but little was left by the time Augustus, her fifth child, was born.

Elkanah's partner removed him neatly and surgically from the firm and shortly thereafter he left Mary Eliza and their children to fend for themselves while he retreated to the hearth of his first wife's daughter Isabella.

No one seems to have minded very much.

Following a tried and true family formula, Mary Eliza opened a boardinghouse, while Charlotte, the eldest, cast about for a quick way to add to the family coffers.

She loathed sewing, abominated housework, had only a rudimentary education, and, at 13 was too young and too plain to attract a wealthy suitor. Having summarily disposed of these "feminine" options, she decided to please herself and make a living from her voice which had been much remarked upon.

Mary Eliza was appalled. The stage! No descendant of one of the first families of New England should display herself upon the stage! Charlotte, as was increasingly her wont, ignored these maternal bleats and proceeded. An old sea-captain friend of her grandfather's, part owner of a piano factory, offered musical advice and lessons, and she obtained several choir positions in local churches to pay her way.

The next five years were marked by Charlotte's recurrent mulishness about her chosen profession, and her mother's obsessive adoration of her younger daughter Susan. Susan was everything Charlotte was not — meek, docile, biddable, and *pretty*. More than just pretty, Susan verged on real beauty, and beside her, her dour older sister looked even plainer.

Charlotte's looks would dog her all her adult life. In her early years, her face was all chin and cheekbones and thin down-curving lips. Even her remarkable eyes which were large, grey and expressive were too bold and prominent. It was a face made to play to the second balcony, but it wasn't easy to look at in the mirror. As she grew older and more famous, reviewers ceased to call her "ugly." They substituted "impressive," "handsome," even "dignified" and "majestic." But no one ever called Charlotte pretty, and it was the one thing even *her* determination couldn't overcome.[7]

Shortly before her death, an admirer asked, "Miss Cushman, if you could relive your life, is there anything you'd change?"

Wistfully she replied, "Yes. I'd be a pretty woman. They have life so much easier."[8]

Certainly Susan's life was very *different* from her ugly older sister's. Whether it was easier is questionable.

At 18, Charlotte was certain that she was as ready as she ever would be to take her place on the American operatic stage. Her first big break came when Mary Ann Woods, then an established singer, hired her to perform duets with her as entr'acte music.[9] This was customary. The touring stars felt that it made a good audience draw to have a local "talent" appear with them. Most sang once or twice and then disappeared, spending the rest of their lives telling stories about their brief "stardom."

Charlotte, of course, was different. For one thing, all those lessons and all those choir solos had honed and polished her natural talents. For another, she was very eager to learn and very determined to do so. Charlotte quickly moved from duets to a *real* part, appearing as Countess Almaviva in *Figaro* in Boston in 1835.[10] She won immediate favor.

Mary Ann Woods recommended her to Clara Fisher Maeder and her husband who were putting together a company to open a theatre in New Orleans. Charlotte's performance as the Countess was a "trial run" with the Maeders, and they invited her to go south with them.

The trip was disastrous. It began badly. Charlotte and Mary Eliza argued incessantly about the propriety of the venture. Mary Eliza cited increasingly lurid tales of the depravity of the theatre and Charlotte countered with dreams of fame and money. Possibly her mother's protests even acted as a spur for Charlotte's ambitions, for few headstrong 18-year-olds can wait to meet depravity face-to-face.

When the Maeders left Boston, Charlotte went with them. The journey south was arduous and physically taxing even for a healthy young woman, and when they arrived, bad news awaited them — the theatre was unfinished. Despite this setback, performance dates were announced and the company began rehearsal in the Hall. The plaster was still damp and carpenters labored to finish the interior walls. The racket was deafening.

The theatre was the largest opera house America had ever seen, rivaling the great houses of Naples and Milan. Certainly Charlotte had never seen so cavernous a space.

Day after day, Charlotte, fighting loneliness, throat problems, and the sickening feeling that her mother might have been right after all, rehearsed valiantly. When the troupe opened, she sang a familiar role, Countess Almaviva, badly. Most reviewers charitably ignored her. Others mentioned her briefly — "inaudible," "untrained," and "untalented" were the kindest of her notices.[11]

Despite the dreadful mentions, she continued to perform until she no longer could. A nightmare engulfed her. Every singer fears losing her voice, even for a few days. Charlotte's disappeared permanently. Whether it was stress, dampness, the climate, or simple maturity and bad training, Charlotte had to admit that her high notes were screeches and her low ones, growls. In between she cackled.

Her fledgling career as an opera singer was finished.

Simple stubbornness and the kindness of the Maeders who continued to cast her in small nonsinging roles were all that stood between her and an ignominious journey back to Boston and Mary Eliza's tongue.

James Caldwell, the former actor who owned the theatre, seeing her plight, advised her to try the dramatic stage, discerning in the raw power of her distress something "theatrical."[12] He sent her to James Barton, a local actor who had grandiosely announced a production of *Macbeth* without a leading lady in sight. Barton needed a Lady Macbeth and Charlotte needed a job. It was a match made in desperation.

Barton rehearsed her whenever she wasn't spear-carrying for the Maeders. He spent most of the rest of his time in deep depressions. Charlotte knew the *words* all right, but her prim New England upbringing stood between her and any emotional displays (i.e., acting). Barton had nearly despaired of banishing seven generations of Cushman ghosts, and the more recent imprint of Mary Eliza's strict teachings. Reluctantly he told Charlotte he was looking elsewhere for his murderous damsel.

Charlotte lost her temper. So did Barton. The scene rapidly degenerated into a loud, vulgar, emotion-packed brawl with name-calling and invective on both sides.

Picture a scene from a forties movie — the director of a play hurls insults at the ladylike young ingenue. She responds in kind. Halfway through her outburst he calls out, "That's *it*. You've GOT it! Now play the scene just *that* way!!" — end of crisis — on to stardom in a hit. . . .

It happened precisely the same way in New Orleans in 1835. Barton, having raised Charlotte's emotional temperature, kept her as Lady Macbeth, and audiences applauded the novice again and again.[13]

Only one other event threatened to mar Charlotte's dramatic debut. It seems to have escaped the notice of both Barton and the young actress that she lacked the wardrobe for the role. The morning of her performance she confessed to Caldwell that she had literally "nothing to wear." In those days theatres didn't keep stocks of costumes, as actors were supposed to supply their own. Caldwell finally sent her across town to the St. Charles Theatre where *Macbeth* had recently been presented in French. There she met Madame Clozel who had played the role. Clozel was quite short and very rotund, sporting a 72-inch waist. Her heart was as big as her girth, however, for she not only agreed to lend Charlotte her costume but pitched in and spent the afternoon doing the alterations necessary to adapt it to Charlotte's tall, slender build. Madame sent her on her way with a much-tucked and disguised costume and warm wishes for her debut. Perhaps the costume was lucky for Charlotte. Certainly she was well received when she wore it.[14]

After *Macbeth* Charlotte was a genuine, certified, leading lady with the notices to prove it. She never looked back.

Despite the glowing reviews, there was little work in New Orleans and Charlotte decided to travel to New York, the emerging theatrical center. Rather grandly, she sent letters to the major theatrical managers there offering her services as a leading lady, and enclosing press clippings of her recent triumphs. No one replied. Somewhat chastened, but convinced that even playing secondary roles in New York was better than starring in sweltering, plague-infested New Orleans, Charlotte, like many another theatrical hopeful, headed to Gotham.

There she was quickly disillusioned. One manager laughed at her outright. Another told her point blank that her looks were against her.[15] Most simply refused to see her. Her search for employment became desperate. Mary Eliza and her brothers and sister were waiting in Boston for the money she faithfully sent home, and New York, even then, was expensive.

Finally T.S. Hamblin, the manager of the Bowery Theatre, engaged her as a "walking lady" or utility player. It wasn't stardom, and the Bowery Theatre, like the neighborhood from which it took its name, was rapidly going downhill. But the money was the best young Charlotte had ever seen ($20 a week), and the manager was willing to advance the $150 she needed to supply a wardrobe for her roles.[16]

Greatly excited, she wrote to Mary Eliza immediately to give up the boardinghouse and bring Charlie, Susan and Gus to New York to live. Charlotte had assumed the role of family breadwinner.

Mary Eliza was eager to end the separation from her daughter and even more willing to abandon the drudgery of the boardinghouse. She was overjoyed to take the boys to Manhattan. Susan, however, was different.

Much as she hated being parted from the girl, Mary Eliza loathed the idea of bringing her to New York and exposing her to the corrupting air of the theatre more. Perhaps she *believed* the tales of depravity she had recited to Charlotte. In any case she regarded it as unthinkable to bring Susan, a nubile 14 year old, to the city. Instead, the child was sent to live with her half-sister Isabella who had also taken in Elkanah.

No doubt Isabella meant well, but when N.M. Merriman, an elderly crony of her father, began to take an interest in Susan, she encouraged him. Merriman was a wealthy 70 year old, not in the best of health, who was entranced by young Susan. First he offered to assume all financial responsibility for the girl's education, then to adopt her.

Mary Eliza was grateful for the financial help but indignantly refused to consider adoption. Then Merriman fell ill. On his deathbed he made a startling proposal. He wished to leave Susan all his money. To do this legitimately, without protests from his family, he suggested a form of marriage.

Isabella urged the match, Mary Eliza wavered and Susan cried. At last though, the prospect of a wealthy widowhood for her favorite swayed Mary Eliza and the marriage was made. Almost immediately Merriman began to recover. Susan soon found herself a most reluctant 14-year-old bride, rather than an exultant, very young widow.

Then things got worse. Merriman left on a "business trip" to New York. When his child-wife opened the door to callers the next day, she found an angry mob of creditors on her doorstep. Her husband had decamped, leaving behind nothing but bad debts.

Mary Eliza's scheme had gone badly awry. No sooner had she received Susan's letter telling of her sudden poverty than another arrived. In this one, Susan wailed the worst news yet—she was pregnant!

This, like all their other recent troubles, Mary Eliza blamed on Charlotte's career. Charlotte, meanwhile, scraped together the money for Susan's fare to Albany.

The Cushmans were in Albany because Charlotte's appearances in Manhattan had been abruptly curtailed when the Bowery Theatre burned one week after her engagement. Her unpaid-for wardrobe also went up in flames.

In debt, with her family due momentarily, Charlotte took the first job she could find—as a walking lady with the Pearl Theatre Company of

Albany. Mary Eliza and the boys arrived in New York City and were rerouted to Albany. Despite the fact that the Pearl had been the proverbial any-port-in-a-storm, the company there provided the training and seasoning Charlotte needed to hone and define the raw emotional talents Barton had roused in New Orleans.

She and Mary Eliza found lodgings, Charlie took a job clerking, and Gus was sent to school. Charlotte played a dazzling variety of roles, ranging from comedy to melodrama. Here she even took her first boy's part when a member of the company fell ill just before curtain.[17]

In addition to the resident company, the Pearl management frequently engaged traveling stars. Edwin Forrest (who had debuted there) and Junius Brutus Booth were among the established performers who acted opposite the fledgling Miss Cushman. She studied each performance, learning subtleties of style and diction, and not least, how to cope with an old scene-stealer like Booth. Forrest was a particular favorite, as was Mary Ann Duff. Charlotte studied Thomas Cooper and Mrs. Powell, whose performances were reminiscent of the ponderous Kemble-Siddon's "pose and pronounce" school, and to the end of her career, she never quite shook off the enormous stage dignity she absorbed from watching them.[18] Charlotte was aware of the gaps in her stage knowledge and even when she wasn't performing she watched from the wings or the house, studying, learning, memorizing. She knew instinctively *when* something worked, and after months of observation and rehearsal she had mastered both *why* and *how* as well. By the end of her engagement in Albany, she was able to match the Forrests, Duffs, and Booths word for word, gesture for gesture, and effect for effect.

To Mary Eliza's relief, Albany offered another form of rehearsal as well. The theatrical season coincided with the legislative session and the theatre company often hobnobbed with the lawmakers. To everyone's surprise, Charlotte became a belle for the first time in her life.

The Babbitts, Mary Eliza's family, were distantly related to New York governor William L. Marcy, and this was all the social entrée necessary. Charlotte, heady with her stage successes and, perhaps, acting a little off-stage as well as on, flirted and conversed, danced and laughed her way through the season. She broke a few hearts and indulged in her own girlish romance. The gentleman's intentions proved to be less than honorable, so she resolutely turned him away.

Soon the delicate tears of romance were supplanted by the sobs of grief. Augustus, Charlotte's youngest brother and her favorite, was attending school near Albany. For his birthday, Charlotte, with money plentiful for the first time, gave him his heart's desire — a spirited, black riding horse. Gus loved the animal and rode him at every opportunity. During the winter, he and one of his teachers set off for an outing in Vermont. They were cantering along when Gus' horse broke loose, reared and flung the boy onto his head. A farmer who witnessed the incident, rushed to the boy and found him already dead.

Charlotte was distraught. Gus had been her hope for the future. He was, in her opinion, the brightest and best of all the Cushmans,[19] and a desire to rescue him from the debilitating effects of grinding poverty and provide all the schooling his agile brain could absorb, was one of the reasons she was pursuing a career on the stage.

The boy was temporarily entombed in Albany and Charlotte threw herself into her work, assuaging her grief in memorable appearances. She kept the jacket young Gus had been wearing when he died and carried it, carefully wrapped, with her the remainder of her life.[20] Perhaps it served as a reminder never to love too completely again.

Charlotte truly came of age in Albany, experiencing success and tribulation, joy and failure, and by the close of the season she knew that she was ready for a professional career and New York as she had not been before.

She played brief engagements in Boston and at the National before joining the Park Theatre. The Park was the major house in New York in 1837 and its company was the most prestigious assemblage in the city. It was also the hardest working, performing in constant rep, often rehearsing two plays daily while performing a third. The actors were continually exhausted, but the company had the most consistent raves in town. Charlotte had again written Edmund Simpson for a position and this time he replied. Her reputation was growing. Simpson offered not leading roles, but a walking lady's position at $18 a week.[21] The money was less than she'd hoped for, but the chance to play the Park was too good to pass up. The Cushman entourage returned to New York City. This time there would be no abrupt flights to Albany and beyond.

Charlotte made her debut on August 26, 1837, as Patrick in *The Poor Soldier*.[22] She spent three busy, productive years at the Park completing the theatrical education begun in New Orleans and Albany. Her talent won her larger and larger roles and it was at the Park that she first played Meg Merrilies, a role associated with her until her death. There was an illness and she was assigned the part shortly before curtain. There was little time to learn the lines, let alone create any character. Fortunately, the old hag does not appear until the last 20 minutes of the play.

There are many stories, most of which conflict, about that first performance. Charlotte's own recollections, which were perhaps apocryphal, attribute her characterization to a blinding flash of revelation. The script calls for Meg to lurk in a tent and then make a sudden appearance. While duly lurking, Charlotte heard the words which, she said, revealed the gypsy's soul:

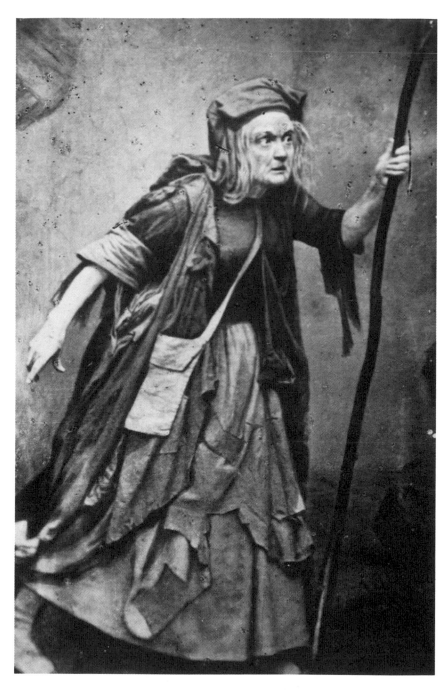

Charlotte Cushman as "Meg Merrilies"

This moor, ye must know, is not in great reputation. There's thieves and gypsies haunt it ... there's an old woman, Meg Merrilies, the queen of 'em, that deals wi' the devil, they say, and can make 'em do anything, if she but lifts up her finger."

"What does Meg Merrilies say; she, whom we must all obey?"

"She say! Why, she *doats*; ..."[23]

Suddenly, with the words "she doats,"[24] Charlotte saw the character whole and complete.[25] Legend has it that her "doating" performance terrified the actors performing with her that night.[26] Whatever the truth of the matter. Meg Merrilies, verging on madness, driven by grief and sorrow, and frightening actors and audiences alike, transformed Charlotte Cushman into a star.

Even before that memorable night, Charlotte had risen steadily through the ranks at the theatre, performing opposite the likes of Forrest and even William Charles Macready, the famous English actor. Macready was something of a snob, professing dislike for the American barbarians, while eagerly pocketing their gelt. It was this attitude that would eventually contribute to the Astor Place riots.

In Charlotte, however, he found something to respect. Her style was old-fashioned to his eyes, harking back to Sarah Siddon and her family. But to his delighted surprise she was willing and even eager to incorporate his own, more realistic approach into the Siddons' stateliness which had, heretofore, been her trademark. Macready confided to his diary in 1843, "The Miss Cushman who acted Lady Macbeth interested me much. She has to learn her art, but she showed mind and sympathy with me, — a novelty so refreshing to me on the stage."[27] Macready's "naturalism" tempered and improved her performances and provided a polish and ease to her characterizations.

Finally, Charlotte felt herself fully trained. She was no longer a raw talent seeking an emotional outlet, but a seasoned professional able to assume any mask however foreign to her true nature. The years at the Park were good ones marked by increasingly larger roles and better reviews.

The Park was also the solution to another Cushman problem. Susan had had her baby, a strapping boy named Edwin (Ned), and now needed to provide for him. Charlotte, looking at many of the ingenues at the theatre who had little to recommend them, imperiously decided that she could train Susan to be at least as good as "that lot." At least *she* was pretty.

Susan, tired of seeing her older sister garner all the praise and all the beaux, fell in with the plan. The Park management agreed and Susan made her debut as Laura in *The Genosese*, supported by her sister and billed as "a Young Lady."[28] Soon she performed well enough to rate having her name listed in the program and even played some leading roles including Juliet to her sister's Romeo.

Occasionally Charlotte and Susan toured in this production and played in some theatres that barely rated the name. One small house in Trenton, New Jersey, was unable to provide them with any scenery for the play but an old quilt which was to suffice for the balcony scene. The theatre manager held up one side offstage and a call boy from the nearby hotel was recruited to hide behind and hold up the other end. Charlotte had just declaimed, "But hark, what light from yonder window breaks? It is the East and Juliet is the sun," when the boy, bored with his task, stuck his face around the impromptu structure and said plaintively, "Miss Cushman, I got to go. I hear my bell at the Hotel." It brought down the house — and the balcony.[29]

By 1841, Charlotte had had enough of life at the Park. Despite her excellent notices and increasing fame in roles like Nancy Sykes and Meg Merrilies, the management still regarded her as a secondary performer and paid her accordingly. Protests availed her naught and she decided to leave, taking Susan with her. She undertook a position as leading actress and manager (Coad says stage manager)[30] at the Walnut Street Theatre in Philadelphia. It was a bad mistake.

Grimly she stuck it out through 1843, but the years were financially draining and emotionally wrenching. Charlotte was an indifferent manager, having little diplomacy and less tact. Stagehands loathed her and resented taking orders from a woman. Actors found her overbearing and autocratic and audiences disliked her productions and stayed away in droves. The only successful plays featured the Cushman sisters and even Philadelphia had to admit that Charlotte could *act.*

At the close of the season, she gave up the Walnut and never again returned to the "counting-house" side of the theatre. She was exhausted and frustrated. Her career was stymied and she felt that American managers would never give her the artistic respect and financial rewards routinely accorded to even second-rate British "stars."

She had remained in touch with Macready, performing occasionally with him in New York, and finally she decided to take his advice and conquer British theatre. If she wanted the money and prestige of the English stars, then she had to *become* an English star. She settled Mary Eliza and Susan in Philadelphia where Susan had accepted an engagement at another theatre, borrowed money, engaged a 14-year-old free black girl named Sallie Mercer as a maid and set sail for London. Just as she had done at 19, Charlotte was journeying in search of her future.

London eventually proved more hospitable than New Orleans, but the city's initial reception to Miss Cushman was cool to the point of indifference.

Charlotte made her presence known to the London theatre managers, but she rather pointedly did *not* ask for employment. Instead she maintained the polite fiction that she was on holiday. Grandly she waited for their solicitations to "break" the holiday with a brief performance. And waited. And waited. Sallie Mercer was reduced to seeking bargains like the day-old baker's dozens of muffins, which with tea made up most their meals. Charlotte fretted daily as her purse grew smaller and still the longed-for contracts failed to materialize.

Finally Sallie called her attention to a gentleman dithering about on the pavement before their lodgings, waiting for the proper calling hour. Charlotte recognized him as Mr. Maddox, the manager of the Princess Theatre. Her ploy had worked! She received Maddox cordially and after some discussion was persuaded to "interrupt" her holiday with a brief appearance at his theatre. She made her debut as Bianca in Milman's *Fazio* and was then engaged to star opposite Edwin Forrest.[31]

Forrest's reviews were mixed, which he attributed to Macready's machinations. This fueled the rivalry between the two actors. Charlotte must have had a difficult time walking the tightrope of friendship with Macready and Forrest's paranoia.[32] Her performances were universally hailed. London embraced her as a star and theatregoers flocked to see this powerful new actress whose talent and voice were beyond compare. Unbelievably, she was also an American! One critic declared that her debut surpassed anything seen in an English theatre since the brilliance of Edmund Kean 30 years before.[33]

Not since John Payne's *Hamlet* had convinced Londoners that not all "colonists" were Red Indians had there been such a sensation from the other side of the Atlantic. Not even Forrest's debut had been so well received. Charlotte Cushman was the first American woman to be embraced as a major actress in London.[34]

She basked in her glory. Once again she had gambled on herself and once again she'd won. She took a small house in New Bond Street and settled down to make money and enjoy the new-found adulation of the London crowds. She went from triumph to triumph, appearing as Lady Macbeth, Meg Merrilies, Nancy Sykes, Romeo, and Queen Katharine. Each set of reviews was better than the last, and Maddox kept extending her contract.

In London she built the repertoire of roles which defined her stardom. They became her "signature." First among these was Lady Macbeth. She initially appeared in the role in New Orleans and it remained distinctively hers for the next 40 years. Her performance was not subtle. She stalked the stage like a hungry tigress constantly calling for blood and driving Macbeth closer to madness with each gory deed. There is a theory that the "Third Murderer," whose presence and identity have never been satisfactorily explained, was Lady Macbeth herself. Certainly Charlotte's sanguinary lusts gave credence to the idea. Her Lady Macbeth was an elemental force, seeking power and feeding on each ghastly murder. Audiences were terrified, horrified, and entranced. Some critics disagreed with her choices for the role — she once advanced the theory that the Macbeths were drunk when they planned and executed their plot[35] — but none could deny her presence:

> I do not believe her conception was the right one, but the power with which she realized it compelled admiration and wonder. It was melodrama "in excelsis" . . . She was the source and mainspring of the whole tragedy. She was inhuman, incredible, and horribly fascinating.[36]

Small wonder she sometimes found it difficult to persuade actors of the first rank to perform opposite her in "the Scottish play." She often complained that "The actors who come on for Macbeth are usually such *little* men: I have to look down at them."[37] Winter carefully interprets this to refer to both their stature and their presentment of the role. Edwin Booth was one whom she found inadequate, judging his more understated style not up to her own bloodthirsty interpretation.[38] She seems to have been rather hard on the Booths generally, for when John Wilkes Booth played opposite her, she struck him with such force that she opened the stitches on the side of his neck where Dr. Frederick May had recently removed a large tumor. Booth bled copiously and had to return to Dr. May to be patched up. The result left an unmistakable scar which was the main means of identifying Booth's body after his assassination of President Lincoln.[39]

Meg Merrilies in a dramatization of Scott's *Guy Mannering* was equally entrancing, but for different reasons. Someone once remarked that Charlotte Cushman's Meg was what Walter Scott would have written if he'd had any imagination.[40] Certainly her interpretation did not lack verve. "It embodied physical misery, wandering reason, delirious imagination, and the wasted tenderness of a loving but broken heart; and it was tinted with the graphic colors of romance . . . the spectator saw a creature of the ideal world and not of earth."[41] If Lady Macbeth was wicked, Meg was mad. It is the role with which Charlotte was most identified and the play virtually disappeared after her death. No other actress could compare with her evocative portrayal.

Queen Katharine provides a welcome contrast from madness and blood lust. *Henry VIII* was Shakespeare's last play, written in 1613 for a command performance before Nan Bullen's daughter. Small wonder that Katharine is a problematic character. In Charlotte's hands, however, she became the embodiment of womanly dignity and queenly fortitude. Clapp provides us with an eyewitness account of her performance.

> Miss Cushman's impersonation of Queen Katharine . . . must be accounted her crowning achievement, and, therefore, the highest histrionic

work of any American actress ... her Katharine was a document in human flesh, to show how a heavenly minded humility may be a well-spring of dignity, how true womanly sensibility may exalt the queenliness of a sovereign.... It was in the second scene of the fourth act that Miss Cushman's genius and art found their loftiest and most exquisite expression. Katharine ... is led in "sick." ... Nothing of its kind that I have heard surpassed the actress's use of the "sick" tone of voice through all of Katharine's part of the fine dialogue.... Miss Cushman avoided excess with the nicest art, but quietly colored the whole scene with this natural factor of pathos.... The throb and thrill of her voice in the ... lines deserve never to be forgotten. ... After Miss Cushman, all recent attempts, even by clever actresses, to impersonate Katharine of Aragon, seem to me light, petty, and ineffectual.[42]

In later years, she also played Cardinal Wolsey in the same play (though not at the same time), the only woman to enact this role. She garnered less praise for the Cardinal than for the Queen, perhaps because the role allows less opportunity for the play of her "vocal cello." During the 19th century Charlotte's penchant for masculine roles was not the eccentricity it seems now. It was quite the "thing" for women to take male leads, and a number of actresses so displayed their talents. It was all part of the theatrical tradition. Like Mrs. Battersby, Mrs. Bartley, Mrs. Barnes, and Mrs. Shaw,[43] Charlotte played Hamlet, often borrowing the costume from Edwin Booth and cursing him as she struggled into his lean-shanked tights.[44] Booth swore that she played the part to revenge herself on him for performances they'd given in *Macbeth*. "Charlotte is determined to show me how a masculine role is to be played," he joked.[45] If most critics found her performance as Hamlet lacking, they outdid themselves in praising her Romeo: "I witnessed on Wednesday night with astonishment the Romeo of Miss Cushman! Unanimous and lavish as were the encomiums of the London press, I was not prepared for such a triumph of pure genius."[46] It was a role she continued to play throughout her career, even into middle age when she was undeniably stout and full-bosomed, characteristics which her costumes seemed to emphasize rather than disguise. Most of the leading ingenues of the 19th century played opposite her and, although a few initially seem to have had reservations, invariably they and the audiences came to accept Charlotte's version of Shakespeare's masterpiece.

> Throughout it was a triumph, equal to the proudest of those I used to witness years ago, and for which I have looked in vain until now. There is no trick in Miss Cushman's performance. No thought, no interest, no feeling, seems to actuate her, except what might be looked for in Romeo himself, were Romeo reality.[47]

At the beginning of her career Charlotte also played comic roles, notably Lady Gay Spanker in Boucicault's *London Assurance* and Lady Teazle in *School for Scandal*, but as she matured and her theatrical stature increased, she confined herself principally to major tragic roles. Nineteenth century audiences were content with this decision.

William Winter, the critic, defines Charlotte Cushman as an actress:

> Charlotte Cushman knew her powers, and when she was on the stage, she justified, to the fullest extent, the esteem in which they were held, by herself, as well as by others . . . for she left nothing to chance and she made impotent the caprice of all observers. You might resent her dominance and shrink from it, calling it "masculine"; you could not doubt her massive reality nor escape the spell of her imperial presence. She was a tall woman, of large person and of commanding aspect, and in her demeanor, when she was thoroughly aroused, there was an innate grandeur of authority that no sensitive soul could resist.[48]

This, then, was the force which conquered London. In time she grew homesick for her family and the rest of the Cushman tribe crossed the Atlantic to join her. Susan had made a small reputation in Philadelphia and New York, but it was mostly of the "She's a pretty girl. Have you seen her sister act?" sort and nasty rumors were starting to circulate about her private life and her child. Mary Eliza was always happy to share Charlotte's success and Charlie was perfectly willing to exchange one clerk's job for another.

After the initial joy of seeing her family again after so long a time, Charlotte found herself chafing for the first time under the restrictions they placed on her movements and her friends.

The house in New Bond Street had become a salon with its hostess as the charming center of attention. The literati and the bohemians flocked to its doors. She made friends with many of the leading lights of art, literature and music. It was a society which condoned a looser way of living than had been possible in Boston. Charlotte found the attention and praise heaped on her, particularly by her female admirers, exciting. When Mary Eliza arrived, she made it quite clear that she disliked Charlotte's new-found friends, and more particularly, her new way of life.

The exact nature of Charlotte's relationships with Eliza Cooke, Matilda Hays, Emma Stebbins, and other women remains unclear. Rumors abounded. Both Cushman sisters lived in a swirl of gossip, with Susan reputed to be too fond of gentlemen and Charlotte of ladies. Certainly Charlotte added fuel to the rumors by her manner of dressing (frequently assuming a coat, collar, tie, and breeches),[49] by frequently playing masculine parts on stage, and by indulging in what Elizabeth Barrett Browning called "female marriages."[50]

Mary Eliza was unprepared for this public display and after a period of increasing friction between them she left, undertaking to keep house for Charlie who had found another of his innumberable clerk's jobs in London. Charlotte, while regretting the breach, insisted that she be allowed her freedom, including the freedom to be talked about. Mary Eliza continued to be proud of Charlotte's success and dependent on her financially, but she refused to countenance her lifestyle.

Meanwhile Susan, unlike her sister, found "life upon the wicked stage" beginning to pall. Rumors about her morals had traveled across the Atlantic, and, though they were unfounded, caused people to look at her askance. The gentlemen she attracted rarely had marriage in mind, and those that did tended to evaporate when confronted by the solid reality of her young son. In contrast to these suitors, wealthy Englishman James Muspratt was seriousness itself. When he proposed, Susan, true to her Babbitt blood, snapped him up. He provided her with a large home, wealth, children and the chance to retire from the stage. Even *he* wasn't terribly enthusiastic about Ned who had been spoiled by his mother, his aunt, and his grand-mother. In time, Charlotte, who was very fond of the boy, and who, perhaps, envied her sister's domesticity and loving family, resolved the problem by adopting Ned. This arrangement seemed to suit all concerned and Ned remained a devoted "son" the rest of Charlotte's life.

The London years were good ones and she stayed in England for five years before her triumphal return to America. When she did, it was to enor-mous publicity and sold-out houses wherever she appeared. Wemyss called her "the pride and ornament of the American Stage."[51] "Our Charlotte" had stormed the British citadels and, like General Washington, had conquered. American audiences could not get enough of their heroine. She was over-whelmed by the outbursts of patriotic affection she aroused.

True to her New England heritage, Charlotte was also a hard-headed businesswoman who had entered the theatre to support her family. She calculated her worth and the amount she hoped to gain from her American performances and decided on the date on which she could put the theatre behind her and return to the respectable gentility which was her birthright. This had been her goal since the first *Fazio* in London.

As May 15, 1852, approached, Cushmania peaked. Her farewells had been announced and audiences flocked to the theatrical event of the decade, if not the century. Freed at last of the bondage of costumes and half-hour curtain calls, Charlotte retired — not to Boston or London but to Rome, haven of many other artistic souls. There she took a villa and opened her home to other American women seeking free expression.

Mary Eliza would have been appalled at the household. Eventually even Charlotte tired of the petty intrigues and jealousies, but at first she doted on being doted on. She also made herself immensely unpopular with the other expatriates living in Rome by constantly seeking to promote the works produced by her "salon." She worked tirelessly to encourage patrons to purchase the paintings, sculpture, and poetry created by her friends.[52]

By her efforts, Charlotte was seeking to demolish the then current theory that art produced by women was inherently inferior. Always

intense, her fervor in promoting "her" artists led her too far in the opposite
direction. Women's art, she seemed to be declaring, was invariably
superior to the majority of masculine works. As is often the case, the passion she used to state her case rebounded upon her and aroused the wrath
of Rome's (mostly male) artistic community.

In time she recognized that the dramas with which she was surrounding herself were but substitutes for the dramatic life she had abandoned.
Accordingly she announced a limited return to the stage. This love-hate
relationship she had with her profession eventually led her to announce
more farewell performances than anyone, except Bernhardt. It never seemed
to affect the audiences' regard for her, and each time they eagerly attended
her "farewells" as if this time, indeed, they were final.

It was also in Rome that she discovered a lump in her breast. The spectre of cancer had haunted her since childhood when she watched her Granny
Babbitt die by inches. The doctors poked and prodded and solemnly announced the results. A mastectomy was required. Surgery in those early
days of anesthesia[53] was a painful and traumatic affair and many patients
died. Charlotte was months in recovery and then discovered lumps under
her arm.

The remainder of her life was a battle against pain. She played many
engagements, usually appearing in the roles which had made her famous.
The breach between her mother and herself never really healed, although
they were once again united when Susan died[54] unexpectedly after a linger-
ing and inexplicable illness. Susan's death was a profound shock to
Charlotte. There had been a certain rivalry between them and they had
grown apart in adulthood, but Charlotte still felt an intense bond to her
younger sister. Now it was irrevocably severed. This intensified the sadness
she felt over the estrangement from her mother.

At the time of Susan's death, Charlotte was at the top of her profession, internationally acclaimed. She had achieved success largely by her
own efforts. She was proud of her financial independence and her theatrical
reputation. The final decade of her life was an unadulterated series of
triumphs marred only by the constant worry of cancer and her increasing
weakness as the disease took its toll. At her final performance, shortly
before her death in 1876, a tribute was arranged for America's greatest actress and William Cullen Bryant presented her with a laurel wreath.

When the end came, she died, not of cancer but of a chill, sustained
in the hotel corridor, which turned into pneumonia. Ned was with her and
she was planning a western tour, "when I improve."[55] Charlotte's position
as the first American woman was clearly established. Her passing rated
headlines around the world and two continents mourned. Half a century
later she was inducted into the Hall of Fame, the first member of the
theatrical profession to be so honored. Her public saw her as a symbol of

the stature of the American theatre. The generations of actors who followed her did not need to achieve English fame to validate their careers: "Charlotte Cushman . . . emphasized the fact that we were no longer a province of England."[56] The critical level of performance in the American theatre had been raised to the point where a successful American star was as highly rated as a successful English one. The home-grown American theatre had matured along with its home-grown American star.

To a demonstrable extent, Charlotte Cushman can be held accountable for this growth. Certainly she set a high standard and served as a role model in her career. Young Americans eager for the stage no longer had to look abroad for actors to emulate. The greatest was readily available in an authentic American version. Yet she made no conscious effort, opened no schools, promulgated no techniques. Advice and insight, when offered— which was rarely—were nebulous and difficult to follow. When Mary Anderson came to her for evaluation, Charlotte told her, "Begin at the top. Don't endure the drudgery of small parts in a stock company under the direction of some coarse nature."[57] Not an easy task for a novice. She appeared to be uncomfortable discussing her techniques, and when asked point-blank by Henry Goddard, explained with difficulty, "to project a strong emotion the player must himself feel the emotion—especially if he is an English or American actor." The person of Anglo-Saxon blood, she emphasized, has too much self-consciousness to impress an audience if he does not lose himself in a part. She testified that she felt the passion she assumed in her roles, and her fellow actors agreed that she indeed seemed to live everything that she did on the stage.[58]

Toward the end of her career, it was an open secret among performers that Charlotte would pound on her cancerous breast at the finale of *Guy Mannering* so that the rush of pain would make Meg Merrilies' death shriek more realistic and bloodcurdling. Audiences quivered in their seats, transfixed by the tragedy they were watching, unaware of the gruesome origin of Charlotte's powerful cry.[59]

She had been taught by Macready that painstaking care, illuminated by those flashes which inspired, were essential in the study of a role, and she applied those lessons to the staging of plays in which she appeared, driving actors and management alike mad with her search for perfection through preparation. "At rehearsals she was particular in the utmost detail. She insisted that every movement and gesture and piece of business be worked out before a performance."[60] Thorough and complete rehearsals are thus one of her legacies to the modern theatre. Another, now institutionalized, is the company curtain call. Olive Logan tells how Charlotte hated forcing her way through the narrow opening behind the roller drop to take her individual bows, and so insisted that the curtain be raised and the entire cast be presented for applause.[61]

But Charlotte Cushman's ultimate contribution to the theatre may well be the legend of her greatness. Each succeeding generation of actors is measured by the one which went before, and each seeks to supplant the previous performers in the public's eye and heart, and in the critic's pen. Each generation perpetuates the tradition of the great performances and creates anew the legends. Charlotte Cushman elevated the aspirations of the American actor and may well have inspired the next century of performances. Actors who do not even know her name strive to create characters that will live in the public memory as her Lady Macbeth and Meg Merrilies did. If they are successful some small part of Charlotte's legacy is passed on: "She was not a great actress merely, but she was a great woman.... When she came upon the stage she filled it with the brilliant vitality of her presence."[62]

Act III

THE MANAGERS

Perhaps the most arduous position in the 19th century theatre was that of manager, and it is hard to understand why so many actors aspired to just those difficult duties. To add to the stress, most managers also performed with their companies, often in starring roles. Thus the whole weight of the company rested on their shoulders. There were decisions to make — plays to choose, bills to pay, touring routes to be mapped out, tradesmen to haggle with, taxes and regulations, recalcitrant actors, scenery, costumes and playwrights to be dealt with.

For most of the 19th century rampant Victorianism persisted, which regarded women as "the fairer sex" and especially "the weaker sex," despite all evidence to the contrary. The theatre, out of necessity, admitted egalitarianism of endeavor, but even there, prevailing legal, social and moral conditions created conformity with this view of "the little lady." Thus it is all the more remarkable that Laura Keene and Mrs. John Drew were able to overcome these notions and prove their worth as managers in an age when such notions were perverse and decidely not the norm.

To be sure, neither was an ideal manager. Laura Keene was idiosyncratic and imperious to a fault, and Mrs. John Drew, though demanding of her company, put her family first in arranging the distribution of roles, sometimes to the detriment of the ensemble.

It is tempting to view these very "modern" women as 20th century businesswomen and to see them as heroines of a "cause," but they are most impressive when viewed in their own right and within the context of their own century.

Their achievements, laudable in themselves, are even more so when compared with those of their contemporaries. Both women's companies were financially successful and both challenged prevailing artistic standards. Laura Keene's died prematurely, and Mrs. John Drew's outlived its era and eventually succumbed to "modernism" and a change in popular taste, but in their heyday both women successfully overcame the masculine dominance of theatrical management and were followed by other women, some successful, some not. The closed door was now not only ajar, but invitingly wide open.

Laura Keene

The date was April 14, 1865. The place, Washington, D.C. A newly reunited nation was enjoying the early spring and attempting to heal the breaches in society caused by four long years of war. It was time to mourn the dead and celebrate the living; to weep in privacy and laugh in public.

The theatres, often shuttered during the recent conflict, had reopened with a flourish. Most of the bills featured comedies. Their audiences sought the healing solace of merriment.

Our American Cousin, featuring the splendid antics of Harry Hawkes, clown consummate, as Asa Trenchard, had announced the final performance. It was to be a benefit for Laura Keene in her one thousandth appearance as Florence Trenchard. The late editions of the *Washington Evening Star* carried the news that, like his constituents, President Lincoln needed to put sorrow behind him, and would attend the evening's production.

The night which began so lightheartedly ended in a tragedy that would echo down the years, leaving in its wake madness and death.

Each of the people most intimately concerned with that night's dreadful deeds found his or her life irrevocably marked by the devastating events of the soft April evening. Murky black ripples of contamination spread wider and ever wider — to an innocent doctor in Maryland[1]; to the greatest living American actor[2]; to a drunken Army sergeant[3]; and to the entire theatrical profession.[4]

The finger of suspicion rested squarely for a time on the troupe performing at Ford's Theatre that night. It is easy to understand the logic of that suspicion, less easy to forgive its aftermath.

The audience that evening was delighted with the performance they were watching. High above the stage in a specially reserved box, a tall, thin, saturnine man shifted in his seat and glanced sideways at the rapt concentration of his companions. Even the foolery of the popular comedy couldn't totally distract him from the workload that awaited his return to his desk. The need to make unpopular decisions worried and wearied him.

"Asa Trenchard" had just declared, "Well, I guess I know enough to turn you inside out, old gal — you sockdologizing old man trap!"[5] and the theatre rocked with laughter as the door in the back of Lincoln's booth eased open. The guard who should have been keeping watch was downing whiskies in the bar instead. Later it would be whispered that he bought drinks with money given him by Mary Lincoln. A slender, handsome, frustrated, disturbed actor slipped into the darkened theatre box and carefully drew aim with a small pistol. He held the .44 derringer to Abraham Lincoln's head and fired once at point-black range. The shot that rang out ruined the hopes of a nation, drove a woman to madness,[6] made the name "Booth" anathema to America, and nearly destroyed the career of Laura Keene, America's first woman theatre manager. Before Colonel Rapp, also in the box, could grapple with him, Booth leaped to the stage, crying "Sic semper tyrannis!" It was a moment of high drama and the actors onstage and in the wings were shocked into immobility. Later, they would be criticized and called co-conspirators for their failure to halt John Wilkes Booth's escape.

Booth had counted on his familiarity with the theatre to facilitate his getaway. Only two flaws marred his carefully thought-out plot to redress the wrongs suffered by the Confederacy. At the last moment, General Ulysses S. Grant, bane of the South, cancelled his plans to go to *Our American Cousin* that evening, and thus narrowly escaped Booth's bullets,[7] and Booth, in his dramatic leap from the Lincoln box, injured his leg.

Nonetheless, he managed to evade capture in the capital, and escape south to the recently conquered lands which he expected to rise as one and hail him as their deliverer. Instead he rode straight to his death.[8]

His only legacy was a shattering suspicion of the entire theatrical profession. Guilt by association weighed most heavily on his brother Edwin, who was driven from the stage and who spent years regaining his lost reputation and denying involvement in his younger brother's Confederate dreams, and on Laura Keene, manager of the company which was performing that night.

Laura Keene was a brilliant English actress who had spent most of her career in the United States. She left England in 1852 at the urging of Lester Wallack who was looking for a fresh, exciting actress to star at his American theatre. When Wallack saw her as Paulina in *The Lady of Lyons*, he was instantly smitten. She had a graceful carriage, striking dark auburn hair, creamy skin, and large, entrancingly dark eyes.[9] All this and she could remember her lines too!

The lady whom Wallack imported to headline at his Lyceum on the corner of Broome and Broadway was no novice in the theatre. Her early years are cloaked in secrecy and little is known of her upbringing. However, it seems quite certain that she was born in London. Her family name *might* have been Lee,[10] and her father *might* have been an upholsterer or draper. She was born variously in 1820,[11] 1826,[12] or 1830.[13] One suspects that she might have lopped a decade off to make more probable her innocent ingenues to the credulous Americans.

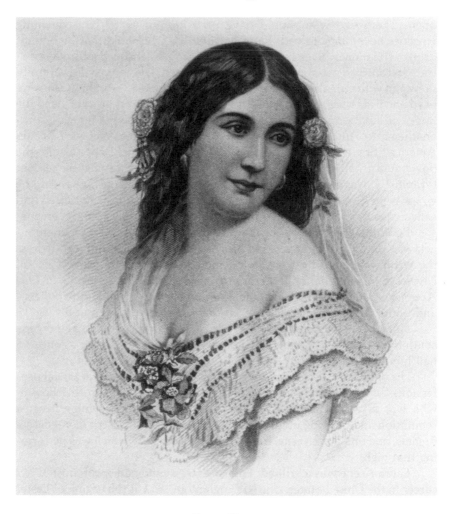

Laura Keene

"When still a girl," the great Rachel "performed so near to her home, her voice could be heard,"[14] and Laura attributed her fascination with the stage to this event. Rachel debuted in London in 1841 and played there again in 1842,[15] so the budding thespian may have been a child of 11 or an impressionable woman of 21. The latter seems more likely, particularly when contemporaries could detect Rachelesque inflections in the Keene style. At roughly the same period Laura came under the influence of the inimitable Madame Vestris.

Madame Vestris was a former dancer and the redoubtable Italian manager of several theatres in London. After the Licensing Act of 1837 was passed, she was allowed to produce a variety of dramas and comedies at her theatre. She was particularly interested in the antiquarian movement and worked with scenic designers to create the "box set" to give her plays authentic backgrounds. She is often credited with introducing modern concepts of the function of scenery to the stage.

Laura seems to have spent some time as a member of the company which Mme. Vestris assembled after her abortive tour of America. Certainly *The Lady of Lyons* from which Wallack plucked his new star was supposed to have been a Vestris production at the Olympic.[16] Hornblow calls this her "debut" performance,[17] but the likelihood is that she had spent several years refining her art before being entrusted with such an important role.

There is an entire alternative story of her antecedents as well. It places her beginnings somewhat lower on the social scale. According to an account gratuitously provided to the *Dramatic Mirror* by an anonymous contributor, Laura Keene was raised in a tavern where she served as a barmaid and was known familiarly to the patrons as "Red Laura." She was married at 16 to John Taylor who apparently expected her to be a similar draw at his own pub. Supposedly she refused, and the marriage soured.[18]

Probably the truth lies somewhere between the sanitized, saintly portrait created by her biographer, Creahan, and endorsed by William Winter, and the muckraking vision of a coarse, ale-pulling, tavern wench offered by her detractors.

This dichotomy in her biography is typical of the dual nature of the woman. Her contemporaries repeatedly extolled the soft-voiced, sensitive actress who threw her very being into her stage work in her company, and in the next breath called her a virago, raging like a fishwife if crossed in her demands. Laura Keene seemed possessed of a vision, and insistent that it assume reality. Perhaps her earliest vision was of her own stage career.

Whether she was the gently born daughter of a middle class tradesman or the main attraction of a pub of brawling drunkards, it was equally unlikely that she would find her way into the company of that unusual ex-dancer turned manager, Lucia Bartolozzi Vestris. And her association with Mme. Vestris is the single solid fact which can be sifted from the deliberately obscured mysteries of her early life.

Mme. Vestris and her revolutionary production style remained a pervasive influence on Laura Keene for the rest of her life. She adopted other, less attractive, habits from Madame too, particularly the autocracy which pervaded her own managerial style.

She left England in 1852, presumably with Mme. Vestris' blessing, and sailed to New York. Except for a brief visit home in 1869, she left London behind her forever, and certainly she never performed there again. Her brief, brilliant career in the Old World was done. Stardom in America loomed on the horizon.

The entourage which sailed on the strength of Wallack's impressive offer included her husband, her mother, and two daughters, Clara and Emma, who were always passed off as her nieces. Her marriage was "unfortunate and unhappy and domestic unhappiness naturally embitters the mind, and often the heart."[19] Thus William Winter, the commentator on things theatrical in the 19th century, attributed many of her less pleasant mannerisms to "untranquil domesticity." That husband's name was John Taylor (which substantiated, however slimly, the *Mirror's* account of her early life), and she eventually shed him through divorce, desertion, or death, sometime in the 1850s, and in 1860 wed John Lutz. Like many other "facts" in her life, this marriage and the "divorce" which made it possible are speculative. She may merely have lived with Lutz. Most accounts call him her "gambler lover" and only Creahan, who wrote her biography at the behest of her daughters, is adamant that the union was legalized. Of course, Creahan had access to private information as well, and may actually have seen the marriage papers.

Lutz seems to have been a rather cruder type. Joseph Jefferson, an actor who appeared with Laura Keene in the original production of *Our American Cousin,* implies that he had no knowledge of the theatre. "Here was a rough man, having no dramatic experience, but gifted with keen practical sense, who discovered at a glance an effective play, the merits of which had escaped the vigilance of older, and one would have supposed, better judges."[20] Winter says that "he was not precisely a 'Grandison' but he was sensible and kind and a shrewd business manager."[21] Lutz may have been a shrewd businessman *and* her husband, but even he was "brushed aside"[22] when Laura Keene's famous, imperious, impetuous temper took hold.

It may have been this impetuosity which led her to leave Wallack's employ after a comparatively short run. She made her debut as Albina Mandeville in *The Will* by Frederick Reynolds on September 20, 1852, and was an immediate success.[23] She continued to play a rather standard run of Shakespearean heroines — Beatrice, Rosalind, et al. — and the other popular plays of the day, including, as always, Pauline in *The Lady of Lyons.* She received excellent notices, but these seem rather to have gone to her head. Within months she had determined to star under her own management. Despite Wallack's protests she was adamant. She left the Lyceum abruptly, sending word to the theatre that she would not appear that evening. It arrived moments before the curtain was to rise on *The Rivals.* Fortunately there was another actress, Lydia Languish, who could play her role and the performance continued, but Wallack was furious.[24]

Soon the Keene-Taylor household was on the move again — this time to Baltimore where she opened a theatre and failed almost immediately.

How Wallack must have chortled when *that* news filtered back to New York. From Baltimore she "wandered West,"[25] playing as she could with various companies until she fetched up in San Francisco in 1854, doubtless much wiser in the ways of the American psyche and the American theatre. In San Francisco she was engaged to play opposite young Edwin Booth. Initially she and Booth did not get along and her notices were not what she expected. Booth, the son of legendary actor and drinker Junius Brutus Booth, had learned the business at his father's knee and found laughable and unnecessary the preparation which Laura brought to her roles. For her part, she found Booth's irreverence for his profession unsettling. Characteristically, she blamed Booth exclusively for their lukewarm reception. For his part, he quipped that "he felt it Keenely."[26]

Despite her misgivings about their disparate performing styles, she agreed to an Australian tour in 1854. She may have had another motive which overrode her theatrical common sense. Her rocky marriage to John Taylor had broken down completely. Except for his demands for money, she never heard from him. There were rumors that he had drifted to Australia and died there, and Laura wanted to be very certain that he would trouble her no more. Australia defeated her. Her searches there proved inconclusive. John Taylor, living or dead, wasn't to be found anywhere she looked while on tour.[27] She probably had to go through a form of divorce prior to her second marriage in 1860. Her personal concerns may have been unresolvable, but when the Australian tour was concluded, she returned to New York trailing clouds of Outback glory and took over the Metropolitan Theatre, which she renamed "Laura Keene's Varieties" in November 1855.[28] Surprisingly, the theatre was a success and when she lost the building to William Burton in a legal wrangle the following year, she was able to raise a public subscription to build a new theatre on Broadway between Houston and Bleecker streets.[29] For the next eight years, "Laura Keene's Theatre" was one of the most popular houses in town.

"The first actress in this country to enter the managerial field,"[30] Laura Keene had learned a great deal during the years between the Baltimore fiasco and the New York success. She modeled her productions after those of her mentor, Mme. Vestris, whose style had not become popular yet on this side of the Atlantic. Vestris and Keene were of the new "realistic" school. If a production called for a Louis XV settee, she did not fob the audience off with a Queen Anne sofa. The settee was either a genuine antique, or as close to authentic as could be found. Laura Keene's productions became bywords of exactitude and authenticity. In addition to managing the theatre and directing the productions she starred in the majority of the plays, oversaw the scenery, and designed many of the costumes.

Sometimes things didn't go exactly as she had planned and crises arose.

Kate Reignolds, a devoted member of the company, remembered one such performance.

> One night when *Much Ado About Nothing* was to be given, it was found, almost at the last minute, that the costumes were not ready. All the women not in the cast were pressed into service. Under Laura Keene's direction the unfinished garments were sewn upon the wearers. The time running short, the distracted manager, who had her own hands full and was yet to dress for Beatrice, called all the lords and attendants to stand before her, and sending to the paint room for a pot and brush, finished the borders of the "jackets and trunks" in black paint! "Now keep apart! Don't sit down! Don't come near the ladies!" with her spasmodic quick speech and she was off to array herself in a twinkling for the dainty young lady of Messina.[31]

Laura Keene's repertoire included over 150 roles and some of the plays were so popular that they enjoyed relatively long runs, which was an uncommon occurrence in the 1850s and 1860s. She played Florence Trenchard in *Our American Cousin* 1,000 times during the course of her career, commencing with a run of six months at her own theatre when she initially produced it. She was a remarkable woman who made a tremendous impact on those who encountered her. William Winter remembered her clearly:

> There is a kind of woman who inspires at once sympathy and a cautious reserve. In appearance she is almost seraphic; in temperament, severe. All that I saw and heard of Laura Keene, when she was managing her theatre in New York . . . caused me to consider her a woman of that kind. By the members of her theatrical company, over whom she ruled with imperious, sometimes even arrogant, authority, she was called "The Duchess." There is a way of government which maintains dominance and obtains obedience without wounding the pride or hurting the feelings of anybody who may happen to be in a subservient position. That was not the way of Laura Keene, who looked like an angel, but was, in fact, a martinet. You could not help liking her, and at the same time you could not escape the intuition that she was a person of impetuous and fiery temper. But she was a remarkable figure on the stage. . . [32]

Critic Winter is candid in his judgment. Until the day of her death, Clara Taylor, one of Laura Keene's daughters, kept a horsewhip by her at all times on the off chance that she might get the opportunity to use it on Mr. Winter.[33]

Not all the actors who appeared in Laura Keene's company would have agreed with Winter, however. Joseph Smith certainly didn't:

> Miss Keene was a very charming woman; kind, gentle, generous, and considerate to her actors. I was connected with her theatre in California and also with her theatres in New York. As a business woman and a manager she had no equal. Her plays were produced with an artistic and financial spendor practically unknown at any other theatre in her day. As an actress she was equally great in every part. . . . As her pathos came

from the heart, it touched the hearts of her audience. Laura Keene lived before her day, and was more than loved by the members of her profession who knew her.[34]

Again we confront the duality of her nature. To Winter, she was impetuous, quick to anger, dictatorial and apparently disorganized. To Smith she showed her compassionate nature. Yet actor Joseph Jefferson saw the darker side which Winter wrote about. Many actors emerged from her company stars in their own right. None became more famous than Joseph Jefferson and E.A. Sothern.

Jefferson was a young actor, very impressed to be "on Broadway" — "It was looked upon as a kind of presumption in those days for an American actor to intrude himself into a Broadway theatre; the domestic article seldom aspired to anything higher than the 'Bowery'"[35] — when she first hired him, but he quickly came to know his own worth and he and Laura Keene engaged in a battle of wills.

In his autobiography Jefferson has little good to say of the woman who introduced him to New York audiences. He damns her judgment, belittles her directoral style and accuses her of financial incompetence with equal fluency, even as he acknowledges her unstinting devotion to production values and her talent as an actress and manager.

> Laura Keene's judgment in selecting plays was singularly bad; she invariably allowed herself to be too much influenced by their literary merit or the delicacy of their treatment. If these features were prominent in any of the plays she read, her naturally refined taste would cling to them with such tenacity that no argument but the potent one of public neglect could convince her that she had been misled in producing them. . . . She was most indefatigable in her rehearsals and spared neither time nor pains in planning her effects, but was greatly deficient in system, ... She possessed but slight experience in melodrama, . . . so that when she got into the realm of red-hot conspiracies, blazing haystacks, and rifle balls, she was quite at the mercy of the enemy. . . . Business had fallen off and the theatre was in a fair way to follow in the train of bankruptcy that was dragging everything after it, . . . Laura Keene was both industrious and talented. If she could have afforded it, no expense would have been spared in the production of her plays; but theatrical matters were at a low ebb during the early part of her career, and the memorable panic of 1857 was almost fatal to her.[36]

Jefferson particularly resented her imperious managerial style. The first clash between them occurred during the astounding success of *Our American Cousin* (which Jefferson modestly attributed to his own rising fame), and concerned that other *Cousin* star, E.A. Sothern.

Sothern was a young Englishman who fetched up on American shores, was hired by the Keene Company, and assigned the relatively small and uninteresting part of Lord Dundreary. During rehearsals and early performances he was disconsolate, seeing little opportunity to employ his talents.

However, he eventually threw caution to the winds and began to mug his way through the role, upstaging wildly, creating forever the legendary persona of the "stage Englishman," beloved forerunner to Bertie Wooster. The audiences adored him and the greater the applause, the broader his playing. The theatre began to fill and Laura Keene, while possibly deploring the unsubtle acting, had come too close to financial failure to condemn his lucrative antics. She even conspired with him in further tomfoolery. This is what led to the first confrontation with Jefferson.

She and Sothern had rehearsed a new piece of business, but they'd neglected to tell Jefferson that his cue had been changed. Jefferson entered as he always had and stepped neatly on the new laugh. Laura hissed at him, "Get off the stage and wait for your cue."

"Madame, this *is* my cue," he said loudly.

"Get off, get off!" she exclaimed, while Sothern tugged at his whiskers and capered for the audience to try to cover this all-too-apparent *unstaged* conflict.[37]

When the scene onstage ended, the battle backstage began. Jefferson refused to continue. Laura fired him. Soon most of the company was loudly and heatedly involved. Eventually the impasse was resolved and the play resumed, but the backstage recriminations were prolonged and vituperative. Tempers flared and harsh words were spoken. In time the situation was smoothed over and the incident forgiven if not forgotten. Jefferson continued with the company and, presumably, came in on his new cue.

Sothern continued to pad his part and build his reputation and Lord Dundreary, that inconspicuous, plot-conveying role of the author's intention, continued his crowd-pleasing ways much to Jefferson's evident discomfiture. One suspects a little stage rivalry here—every laugh that Sothern evoked was stolen from Jefferson, the supposed comic relief of the piece, who said,

> Miss Keene was undoubtedly delighted at Sothern's rising fame. I think she found that I was becoming too strong to manage, and naturally felt that his success in rivaling mine would answer as a curb, and so enable her to drive me with more ease and a tighter rein.[38]

However, whatever adjustments were necessary to the egos involved, the audiences rushed to "Laura Keene's Theatre" and brought their money with them:

> As the treasury began to fill, Miss Keene began to twinkle with little brilliants; gradually her splendor increased, until at the end of three months she was ablaze with diamonds. Whether these were new additions to her impoverished stock of jewelery, or the return of old friends that had been parted with in adversity—old friends generally leave us under these circumstances—I cannot say, but possibly the latter.[39]

All the performers in the company benefited similarly, and when the season ended, Jefferson and Sothern were sufficiently well established to be offered starring roles in other companies.

Laura Keene continued in her theatre, producing a string of more-or-less successful plays — often alternating in repertory with the still-popular *Our American Cousin* — until 1863 when she gave up the lease of her theatre and became a touring star.

Several factors may have contributed to this decision. Audiences, and consequently revenues, were falling off as a result of the Civil War, now dragging into its third year. Too, theatrical fashions change nearly as rapidly as the seasons, and what had been innovative and attractive eight years before was now trite and overdone. Her judgment in choosing plays may really have been as poor as Jefferson implied — certainly there were no successes to rival *Our American Cousin* at the box office.

She may simply have been tired. Eight years of constant decision-making, coupled with the necessity to juggle the demands of acting, staging, writing or rewriting scripts to suit her company, weighing financial considerations (even with the assistance of John Lutz, her business manager both before and after their marriage), and creating sets and costumes which suited her purse as well as her own expectations and those of her audiences, may simply have taken a toll.

Whatever the reason, it was not because of the professional incompetence with which Jefferson had charged her. Rather the opposite. She was too concerned and too meticulous and it drained her. An actress who worked with her observed,

> Laura Keene was not only one of the greatest actresses of her day and time, but as a stage manager she had no equal, while she was the greatest business woman I have ever known. Compared with Miss Keene in business, all other women, to me, in the theatrical world, faded into nothing.... She was prompt, precise, punctilious and exacting to the very letter of the law ... but as a manager all other women were mere cyphers or novices compared to her. The mounting of her plays and stage productions was not only on a degree of elegance, unknown and surpassing all other productions then, but has practically been unknown to even elaborate stage productions of today. The lace draperies alone, in one scene of a stage setting under Miss Keene's management would cost hundreds of dollars. Nothing was too expensive for Laura Keene, and nothing but the best ever entered her theatre. She produced one play ... in which one entire stage scene was composed of the finest white lace to be found on the market. Nothing like this scene or stage setting has ever been witnessed on the stage. Theatrical people came to see it, and marveled at the woman's daring as much as the people applauded her wonderful enterprise.[40]

Such attention to detail was exhausting and expensive. If "nothing was too expensive for Laura Keene," running her theatre may have been unprofitable. Then too, there were constant rumors of the closing of the theatres in time of war. She and Lutz might have decided to rid themselves of a potentially disastrous financial entanglement while they still could.

At any rate she began to tour, often appearing in *Our American Cousin*, moving ever closer to that fatal one thousandth performance.

Until the evening when John Wilkes Booth fulfilled his tortured destiny, Laura Keene expected nothing but a future similar to her past. It is true that her popularity was slipping somewhat, but she was still a *star*, and able to draw audiences to every performance. The bullet which killed Lincoln irrevocably killed her career as well. She was waiting in the wings for the end of the scene when Booth leaped to the stage. He pushed past her in his escape, striking her a glancing blow as he passed. Her orchestra leader grappled with him and then fell back, stabbed. The audience at first thought this all a part of the play's action, and then were galvanized by Mrs. Lincoln's shrieks.

When Laura Keene realized what had happened, she left the wings and hurried onstage as the patrons began to rush from the main seating area toward the stage. "Miss Keene, fearing some of them would be injured, or even that a riot might develop, stepped before the footlights and made a plea for order . . . 'For God's sake, have presence of mind, and keep your places, and all will be well' she announced."[41]

She then made her way to the presidential box where she offered or requested to hold Lincoln's head[42]. She knelt on the floor and lifted the wounded man onto her lap. Gradually his lifeblood seeped into her costume, forever staining it.[43]

Curiously, no one attempted to remove her and she spent the remainder of the night with the presidential party. When Lincoln was removed from the theatre to the nearby home of a frightened tailor, she went with Mrs. Lincoln and Clara Harris, who had also been a member of the presidental party, and spent her time comforting the stricken first lady and the grieving girl. Several times during the night she supported Mrs. Lincoln when she made her way to her husband's bedside. Inevitably these moments were accompanied by emotional turmoil and eventually she was roughly told, "Keep that woman out of here!" by the doctors and Secretary Stanton.[44]

The President died before dawn, and the long vigil ended. The body was removed and Laura Keene returned to her lodgings, weary and heartsick. Further shocks were to follow. She, Harry Hawks, and William Witchell, the orchestra leader, had all recognized the assassin as John Wilkes Booth, and though reluctant, were the first to say so publicly.[45] Other members of the theatrical profession at first denied the possibility that Booth could be guilty.

The public had no such qualms, and it was with difficulty that a mob yelling "Burn the theatre," was restrained from doing just that. Given the atmosphere of suspicion in Washington, it is not surprising that Laura Keene and her troupe were arrested for conspiracy the next day.[46] Lutz, who had been acting as a kind of advance man for the tour, returned to Washington at once and was able to secure their release on bond.

The hysteria mounted as Lincoln's body began its final journey and theatrical folk found it expedient to keep a low profile. Even after Booth's capture and death, a residue of suspicion clung to Ford's Theatre and Laura Keene's company and her bookings dwindled.

No longer a sought-after leading lady, she had become somewhat like her old costar Edwin Booth, a theatrical pariah, wandering to increasingly infrequent engagements. So deep was the shame associated with the assassination that William Winter, when he wrote her obituary several years later, said merely, "For a long time after leaving [her] theatre, Miss Keene was unheard of in theatrical life, but it was vaguely known that she was roaming the country with a traveling company. In 1870 . . . she returned to New York. . . ."[47] It seems unlikely that Winter was unfamiliar with her very visible involvement during the assassination, yet it was never mentioned.

Edwin Booth was able to make a comeback, but Laura was too weary, too heartsick, too out of fashion to regain her former stature. She enjoyed a brief vogue as a "lecturer" giving stage readings and then sank most of her remaining capital into a short-lived journal, *The Fine Arts*, "which published at length on the best of paper and with the finest of engraving, articles on such subjects as English painters, art treasures, sculptures, outstanding building, drama, and actors."[48] A favorable mention here marked Edwin Booth's return to the stage. Within the year *The Fine Arts* had folded, taking with it Laura's remaining vitality.

The eight years after Lincoln's death had been marked by a steady decline in her health and her personal and professional fortunes. She felt cursed by the taint of spilled blood and for many years her very real contributions to the theatre were smothered by her involvement in this single sensational act. Laura Keene's true legacy is very different. She was a remarkable artist and an innovative force in the theatre.

One artistic vision guided her company. A single person oversaw the scenery and costumes, selected the plays and conducted the rehearsals. It would be misleading, of course, to view these actions from a 20th-century perspective. The unified and artistic productions at Laura Keene's Theatre bore little resemblance to the concepts of "unity" and "realism" as they are currently defined. In the late 1850s, actors still "possessed parts" which meant that once an actor in a company played the romantic leading role of Romeo, he would continue to play it despite age, corpulence or even a distressing lack of talent, until he left the company or was persuaded to move on to other, perhaps more suitable, types of roles. It was not unusual in smaller companies to see doddering "leading men" of 50 or 60, hamming their way through the role of the love-struck teenager.

Most casting was according to "lines of business." An extension of possessing parts, "lines of business" casting was a handy way of categorizing actors. One might be a "romantic juvenile," a "walking woman," a "utility" man, a "fat character" woman . . . and so forth. Once so designated, actors played all the roles in the company's plays which could be so defined. It was unusual to "break type," and see, for instance, a "singing chambermaid" or soubrette "type" play Juliet. Of course, one company's utility man might be another's romantic lead, and all actors worked assiduously to improve their line of business while avoiding breaking type to a series of lesser roles.

The star was still the main drawing card but, in Laura Keene's company, for the first time in America attention was given to creating unique settings for specific plays.

When Dion Boucicault wrote *The Colleen Bawn*, he sent Laura a set of steel engravings of Ireland, that the scene painters might begin work on drops that suited his yet-unwritten "Irish play":

> My dear Laura:
> I have it! I send you seven steel engravings of scenes around Killarney. Get your scene painter to work on them at once. I also send a book of Irish melodies with those marked I desire Baker to score for the orchestra. I shall read act one of my new Irish play on Friday; we rehearse that while I am writing the second, which will be ready on Monday; and we rehearse the second while I am doing the third. We can get the play out within a fortnight.[49]

The generic sets were gradually being abandoned in favor of specific locales appropriate and even unique to a particular play. Actually, of course, they were still somewhat generic — scenes of the countryside, rather than scenes of so-and-so's pig yard, but they were specifically generic, if such a thing is possible, and suited exclusively for a particular dramatic work. This careful attention to detail was costly and Laura Keene was in the forefront of managers willing to risk profits to create exciting new productions for their audiences. The audiences, hungry for spectacle, were enthusiastic about the changes. Improved production values became good business, but this seems to have been less Laura Keene's motive than a genuine belief in her vision of the theatre "as it ought to be" and her mission to create a sophisticated, elaborate, and artistic theatre. Unfortunately, she was unable to communicate this vision and mission to her contemporaries and their view of her was rather shortsighted. They did not share her grand design, nor were they able to foresee the tremendous impact that this kind of production realism would have upon the theatre for the rest of the 19th and 20th centuries. Instead, their view of Laura was sadly different.

> At the highest she was a clever actress of brilliant comedy; but she wasted her talents, and came at last to be only an experimenter in the hydraulic emotional school. She died of consumption at Montclair, N.J., on November 4, 1873, in her fifty-fourth year. To old playgoers her death was a mournful reminder of time and the rapid extinction of their favorites. In the prime of her beauty and talent, she enjoyed almost boundless favour with the public, but she outlived her popularity and sunk into comparative oblivion; so that the news of her death scarcely caused a ripple of feeling outside of a narrow circle of professional contemporaries and theatrical followers. The moral of her experience was not wholly the evanescence of popularity. Public life may be mutable, but solidity of character and talents do not fail to win for their possessor a place of permanence, at least in the memory of the passing generation. Neither was possessed by Laura Keene and hence her contemporaries scarcely heeded the sound of her passing bell.[50]

This bitter obituary is typical of the view which the 19th century took of her accomplishments.

Much of Laura Keene's life is lost. She deliberately obliterated large sections of her personal experience. Even details of her professional career are dauntingly few. Only her actions remain to be judged. When those actions alone are considered, it can still be said that Laura Keene altered forever the shape of American theatre.

She was a remarkable innovator within the American theatrical scene: "Laura Keene's reputation as an artist was earned and won by her own ability and as such only; achieved at a time in the history of the New York stage when elaborate dramatic criticisms such as are the rule today were entirely unknown...."[51]

She was the first woman in this country to manage a theatre, dealing with financial and production responsibilities at a time when most women couldn't even have pin money except by the gracious dispensation of their fathers and husbands. "Lauded as 'an unexcelled actress' by the *New York Times* (January 12, 1862) and as 'the greatest stage manager I have ever known' by J.H. Stoddard, she was also an innovator. She spent large amounts of money for advertising and in 1867 became the first American manager to encourage native writers by offering one thousand dollars for the best play written by an American."[52]

The mere fact of having been the first actress-manager would be a minor but interesting footnote were it not for the conscious efforts which Laura Keene made to introduce a realistic and cohesive production style at her theatre. Her management career was brief and marred by internal dissents and her own flawed personality, but her far-reaching influence has extended to the modern theatre and almost no other 19th century manager can be said to have equalled the effects of her artistry and expertise.

Louisa Lane Drew

"You had to know how to act . . .
when you went on the stage in those days."
— Fanny Cavendish (The Royal Family)[1]

It was a warm night late in May in 1892. A few carriages rattled past the columns of the old theatre on Arch Street. Inside, the audience, not so large as it had been in years past, applauded enthusiastically when Louisa Lane Drew appeared to take her bow as the Widow Green in *The Love Chase*. Few people in the house that night were aware that they were witnessing the end of an era. Mrs. Drew was withdrawing from the management of the theatre. For 30 years the fortunes of the woman and the building had been bound up together. Their association had lasted even longer, for as a child, newly arrived in America, young Louisa had watched with interest as a new theatre was built in Philadelphia.

Mrs. Drew and the Arch had grown and prospered over the years. Her trips to New York to see new plays and audition actors were like royal processions. Theatre managers hastened to give up their own box seats to her, waiters at Delmonico's vied to serve her table, and critics and performers alike trembled in her presence. As for the Arch, under her auspices, it was the epitome of the well-run theatre, a-gleam with polish and paint, and packed to the rafters with eager audiences.

Now it was all coming to an end.

In 1828, the playbill for the Walnut Street Theatre in Philadelphia advertised the farce *Twelve Precisely* with a cast of five. Amazingly all five characters were performed in a bravura display by Louisa Lane, a seasoned performer, aged eight.

The heir to a theatrical legacy, that by family tradition stretched back to Elizabethan strolling players, Louisa Lane began her career in *Giovanni in London* at 12 months when she was carried on stage by her mother. She was supposed to do what most babies do very well — bawl loudly and make a general ruckus. Instead, she was so entranced by the lights and applause that all she did was coo with delight. It was the last time she would "blow her lines."

Other small roles followed and young Louisa learned to perform as naturally as she learned to toddle: "at the age of five she was sustaining regular roles in melodrama."[2] She spoke her first lines in that grand old melodrama *Meg Murnock; or, The Hag of the Glen*. When she was six, her father, Thomas Lane, died. After a year of small parts and smaller salaries, her mother, Eliza Trenter Lane, decided that life as "a singer of sweet songs and ballads" on the circuit of small English provincial theatres was leading nowhere and that the dangers of life in the former "colonies" might be preferable to starvation in England.

Before they left, Louisa played a final engagement in Liverpool at Cook's Amphitheatre. She played Prince Agib, and appeared opposite a horse, for horses were the principal performers at Cook's. Things went well for most of the run, but on closing night "the horse stumbled . . . and rolled down on to the stage. . . . There was a universal wish on the part of the audience to know if 'the dear little girl was much hurt'; but she was insensible to the kind wishes of the audience, I believe I may truly say, for the first and only time in her career."[3]

Afterwards Louisa and her mother, Eliza, embarked for New York. They sailed on the *Britannia* with nine other actors hired by John Hallam. Details of the period that follow are sketchy. They obtained employment on the circuit that comprised American theatre at that time—first in Philadelphia, where Louisa played the Duke of York to Junius Brutus Booth's King Richard III at the Walnut Street Theatre. Young Louisa was immediately successful. From Philadelphia, she traveled to Baltimore to Joe Cowell's Theatre, where she appeared with Edwin Forrest. Forrest, America's first great native actor, played William Tell, and Louisa was Albert. Edwin Forrest was so entranced with her abilities that, at the close of their engagement, he presented her with an engraved silver medal. She prized that medal all her life.

In 1828, she made her New York debut as Little Pickle at the Bowery Theatre. Afterwards, she performed with all the famous players of her day—Macready, Forrest, Joseph Jefferson III, Tyrone Power, George Holland, and Charlotte Cushman. "Her versatility was extraordinary, allowing her to play in one season, more than forty parts."[4]

Her mother, Mrs. Lane, established a liaison with John Kinlock (or Kinloch), a Philadelphia stage manager whom she married in 1827. A baby was born the following year.

Child actors enjoyed a brief vogue during the late 1820s in America, and Louisa and her mother and stepfather were quick to see the possibilities of a precocious eight-year-old. The effect on the audiences was predictable, and the Kinlocks quickly made a career of managing Louisa while supporting her onstage in small roles. She seems to have made a specialty of playing multiple roles. Besides *Twelve Precisely*, there was *Actress of All Work* (six characters), *Old and Young; or, The Four Mowbrays* (all four Mowbrays), *72 Piccadilly* (five characters) and *Winning a Husband* (seven characters!).[5]

In 1830, as the interest in child actors waned, Kinlock assembled a company and sailed for an ill-fated engagement in the West Indies, then an accepted part of the American "circuit." The voyage was perilous and the ship wrecked. The passengers were stranded for six weeks before a rescue

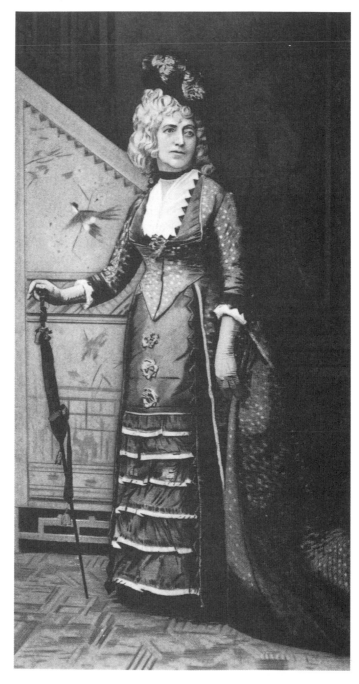

Mrs. John Drew as "Mrs. Malaprop."

could be effected. Presumably they were in mortal danger. Yet Louisa, in her autobiography, admittedly written many years later, treats the period in a curiously light-hearted way.

> When out about ten days we struck a hidden rock — a case of ignorant carelessness I should think, as it was the most beautiful moonlight night. The ship remained standing so everyone got dressed, ready for leaving, as we could, even at night, see the beach before us. The captain found that it was San Domingo. In the morning we all got safely to shore, all our baggage with us; then the crew started erecting tents. . . . Our deck-load had been shingles and staves which proved very useful, as did all the stores from the ship; and we settled ourselves to stay for some time, as they ascertained that we were forty miles from any settlement, and the captain . . . would have to go to the city of San Domingo and obtain a brig to get us off. . . . We were there six weeks and I celebrated my eleventh birthday there.[6]

One suspects that this *very* sophisticated veteran of ten years upon the stage enjoyed the only completely childlike freedom of her girlhood during this traumatic episode.

The company eventually reached its destination and played to great success, but the trip took a heavy toll. Kinlock took ill with a fever, and died, as did the baby. Eliza caught the fever, but managed to survive with Louisa's devoted nursing and the skills of a local doctor. The doctor also discovered that Eliza was pregnant and sent her to the hills for her health. A daughter, Adina, was born. A second daughter, Georgiana, appeared several years later in America. Possibly there was a third, unrecorded marriage.

There was an insurrection and the Kinlocks returned to Kingston. In 1832 they took ship for New York. Louisa's earnings as an actress paid their passage. From this period on, matters worsened considerably.

> New York, April 26, 1832
>
> — To Messrs. Forrest and Duffy
> Gentlemen:
>   Myself and daugher arrived on Sunday last from the West Indies, after a voyage of twenty-two days. I presume it is needless to mention Mr. Kinlock's death, as you have doubtless heard of it long before now. Me and Louisa are at liberty to take an engagement with you. Should there be a vacancy I should be most happy to treat with you — that of first singing or singing chamber-maids — indeed, a general round of business. As to Louisa you are aware what she can do. Your answer by return will oblige your obedient and humble servant,
>
> Eliza Kinlock[7]

Eliza was willing to accept any engagement at all. Unfortunately there was no work at Forrest's Walnut.

Louisa had entered that awkward stage, common to many child actors. Now it is called adolescence; then it was known as unemployment. She was gawky, and her features, maturing from childish innocence, had taken on the full, strong cast of adulthood. She retained, however, her charm and her talent, and Eliza succeeded in obtaining for them a position with the Warren Theatre in Boston. Their joint salary was $16 a week. They obtained a room in the boarding house at the corner of Bowdoin Square and settled down for two happy seasons. "I don't know how we lived," Louisa would recall later. "We had a large room on the second story, a trundle bed which went under the other for the accommodation of the little children, [and] a large closet in which we kept a barrel of ale and all our dresses."[8] During the summers they played with an amateur troupe in Maine and Nova Scotia.

In 1835 the Kinlock family was engaged as part of the troupe for the St. Charles Theatre in New Orleans. Also in the company was Henry Blaine Hunt, late an intimate of George IV, now intent on recouping his fortunes on the American stage. The 45-year-old tenor was entranced with Louisa, 25 years his junior, and her mother was impressed with his connections to nobility. Two months after her sixteenth birthday, they were married. During the second season, the St. Charles instituted Sunday performances. Eliza, a staunch believer, was appalled, and the Kinlock/Hunt ménage moved West. By the time Louisa was 18, she was playing opposite Edwin Forrest in *Macbeth*, in Natchez.

The extended family came East again when Louisa was contracted for a season as the leading lady at the Walnut Street Theatre. How Eliza must have smiled at that irony. Louisa received $20 a week, the highest salary paid to an actress in America at that time. After a year, touring resumed. Louisa was always accompanied by her mother and her half-sisters, Adina and Georgiana, less often by her husband. Ostensibly it was difficult to find managers willing to hire them both, but in truth, the marriage was failing. In 1847 they divorced. Montrose Moses has suggested that perhaps Hunt and Louisa were equally unprepared for the rigors of marriage, he because of his early profligacy, and Louisa because of her youth.[9] Hunt died in New York in February 11, 1854. The divorce, an unusual and scandalous event at that time, does not seem to have harmed her career or to have dimmed the ardors of George Mossop (Moosop), a notorious tippler, whom she married in 1848. His chief charm seems to have been a stammer which disappeared on stage, and when he drank himself to death in Albany, several months later, Louisa appeared more relieved than grieved.

The daring divorcée was thus transformed into a respectable widow. She and her family continued to tour, encountering along the way one John Drew, a handsome Irish character actor. When he came courting her sister Georgiana, Louisa refused his suit on the grounds that Georgiana, nearly 19, was too young to marry! She did not, however, forbid him to call, and two months later, on July 27, 1850, at the age of 30, she married 22-year-old John Drew. Clearly she was a woman who recognized opportunity when it came courting. Kobler described her thusly: "Louisa Lane, in maturity, a somewhat overpowering figure, ample and tending to masculinity, with a blunt chin and nose set in a round face. But intelligence, charm and an air of authority served her as well as beauty when it came to securing a husband."[10]

By contrast, John Drew was not only younger than his bride, he was better looking, with curling brown hair and mischievous eyes. His family had come from Ireland when he was still a boy, so he had been reared in New York, where his father was bookkeeper at Niblo's Theatre. He was a wild youth, shipping out to sea at 13. After several years as a sailor, he returned home and decided to try his hand at acting. He had no training and no theatre was willing to try him out. Eventually he talked himself into small parts with the Richmond Hill Theatre, a quasi-amateur group eager for men. There he learned the rudiments of stage decorum. He followed this with a stint as shopkeeper in Ireland, but managed to get on the wrong side of all the political parties and had to leave. Back in America, he secured a place in a touring company. He excelled in Irish peasant roles, blending pathos and comedy with a hint of sentimentality. Jefferson praised him as an "Irish" actor, noting particularly his ability to "touch the heart ... deeply."[11] Drew played Sir Lucius O'Trigger, Handy Andy, Rory O'More, and with his brother Frank, the Dromios.

The Kinlocks, with the addition of their newest family member, resumed touring. Moses notes, "Mrs. John Drew, once playing in *London Assurance* [in Pittsburgh], created a sensation by having a real carpet and a mirror among the properties for one act."[12] Perhaps this early realism was unsuccessful for it was not noted by the papers for the rest of the tour.

The marriage appears to have been happy and three children were born in rapid succession: Louisa in 1852, John, Jr., in 1853, and Georgiana in 1856. Mrs. John Drew raised a fourth child, Sidney White, of whom Ethel Barrymore said, "[Uncle] Sidney may not have been the son of John Drew, but he was indubitably the son of MRS. John Drew."[13] Kotsilibas, in his biography of Maurice Barrymore, tells the following story:

> It was unusual for Mrs. Drew to fraternize with young members of the company, particularly so to include them in family gatherings, but the handsome young imitator of Dickens was an exception. He spent a great deal of leisure time with his employer. "Robert Craig," she explained, "is one of the most talented young men I have ever met." During the season of 1867–68, Craig was abruptly asked to leave the Arch Street Company. Soon after, Mrs. Drew quit Philadelphia for a long rest in the country. She returned with babe in arms, adopted, she said, and christened him Sidney White. Even when the child grew to be a mirror image of his adoptive mother, no one dared to question. Louisa Lane Drew was above reproach.[14]

John Drew was a talented, handsome actor, very popular with

audiences and his fellows, and with a relaxed, devil-may-care attitude to life. This was very different from Louisa's never-on-a-Sunday upbringing and may have been one of his major attractions for her.

With his growing family even Drew could recognize the need for stability, although Eliza Kinlock, his formidable mother-in-law, no doubt pointed it out on occasion. In 1853 he and William Wheatley took the lease of the Arch Street Theatre. The Kinlocks and the Drews made up a large part of the company and success greeted the venture. Too much domesticity seemed to wear on John Drew's nerves, however, and two years later he threw up the lease to tour England and Ireland. Louisa was furious, and only partially appeased by the fact that Eliza Kinlock was to accompany him. On his return, Drew, prompted by his ambitious wife, reluctantly took up the management of the National Theatre. This venture failed, and the Drews joined the Walnut Street Theatre company. Louisa stayed there the following year, while John went off on a Canadian tour. Unfortunately this only served to increase his wanderlust, and on his return he immediately booked another tour — this time for California and Australia.

Furthermore, he proposed that Georgiana, his never-forgotten first love and sister-in-law, accompany him. Louisa had her misgivings, but when he agreed that their daughter Louisa go along too, she had to consent. John, Georgiana, and Louisa opened to splendid notices in San Francisco and Melbourne. Georgiana even married an actor, John Stephens, whom she met in Australia. This news must have relieved Louisa Lane Drew's worries considerably. However, when they left "Down Under" for England, Georgiana's husband stayed behind to fulfill some engagements. He never caught up with them again, and when they returned to Philadelphia after a three-and-a-half-year absence, Drew arrived with presents for the children, a sheepish expression, and Georgiana's newborn baby in his arms.

Mrs. John Drew, left behind in Philadelphia, assumed the lease of the Arch Street Theatre on August 3, 1861, when the board of directors, inspired by Laura Keene's example, and perhaps despairing of another lessor, offered it to her in lieu of her globe-trotting husband. She accepted after writing for and receiving her husband's permission (John Drew was then playing in Ireland).

The Arch Street Theatre was a venerable Philadelphia institution. Built in 1828, the Arch had been managed by (among others) William Forrest, Edwin Forrest's brother, Francis Wemyss, and W.E. Burton. Coad writes that it "was identified . . . with American drama and dramatists."[15] The "star system" began to break down in the 1850s and this proved to be a boon for the Arch. In 1853, when John Drew and William Wheatley formed a company, it quickly rivaled that at the old Chestnut Street and Walnut Street theatres. After Drew and Wheatley parted company the following season Wheatley soldiered on alone until Mrs. Drew assumed the lease: "she was the first woman in America to enter the field of theatrical management on so large a scale."[16]

It was a risky venture, both for the daring board and the soon-to-be manager. Women in the 1860s were still decades away from suffrage, and a full century removed from the women's rights movement. In this country only Laura Keene had turned from actress to manager, and she was to become a minor victim in a national tragedy.

Fortunately, Mrs. John Drew had only the upheavals of theatrical politics to endure, and although she was eventually forced to succumb to economic pressures and changes in style, she succeeded in running the Arch Street Theatre for 30 years — the first woman in America to become a successful long-term theatre manager.

She proved herself as competent backstage as onstage and as quick to grasp the intricacies of a balance sheet as to memorize the lines for Lady Teazle. Soon the Arch ranked second only to Lester Wallack's theatre in New York. In the beginning she maintained the resident-company system, then predominant in most theatres. The role of managers under such a system was complex, requiring them to serve as director, producer, casting agent, designer, and actor, with side duties as diplomat, financier, and confidant. It was a role Mrs. Drew was destined to play.

It is important to understand the theatrical climate in which she began her fledgling managerial efforts. Prior to 1870 the main producing unit was the resident stock company. Every town of any size had a theatre with a company, and most large cities had two or three. These companies were virtually independent entities. The manager chose the plays to be performed, cast them from the resident actors according to their "lines of business," or hired stars to perform in particular plays, directed them, and saw to the scenery and effects such as they were. Gradually this system broke down as the stars became more and more popular and audiences demanded increasing numbers of them in every production. "Combinations" of stars formed to satisfy this demand, and eventually the combinations became entire touring companies. When this happened, the old repertory way of the theatre died a painful death. It didn't happen all at once — some managers hung onto the old ways long after the audiences had lost interest. Mrs. Drew, for example, didn't give in completely till 1880, and as late as the 1878–79 season, the Walnut Street was still booking individual stars who sent advance men to rehearse the company and then arrived the day of the performance for a quick run-through. Otis Skinner, then a young actor, was a member of the Walnut company and draws this picture of a typical rehearsal:

> One got a general idea of the exits, entrances, and mise en scene, with the injunction to give the star the center of the stage and keep out of his way. A few rehearsals with speeches rattled off, stage business agreed upon, and

we were ready for the performance, leaving the sets, music cues, curtains for the acts, "shouts outside," etc. in the hands of the poor devil of the stage manager, who was sure to let something go wrong, and in consequence be hauled over the coals by the star. First nights were visitations of terror.[17]

The actors of the stock companies frequently had to learn hundreds of lines for a new play when the star arrived with it, and then go on that night with no rehearsal. This led to the practice of tacking up lines in the wings so that they could study the next scene before they played it, and this gave rise to the phrase "winging it," meaning to improvise as needed.

One of Louisa Drew's accomplishments was to impose an order on these slipshod procedures. Rehearsals at her theatre began promptly at 10:00 A.M. She drove up to the theatre in her brougham at five till the hour. The actors rehearsed for the next four hours, sometimes going through two plays at once if there were rapid changes on the bill. The afternoons belonged to the actors for study. Mrs. Drew would go over the books, sign bills, and inspect her theatre to insure that her high standards were being met. An actor who performed in the Arch described it in this manner:

[S]uch immaculate cleanliness from the footlights straight to the building's walls! The floor was scrubbed to a creamy purity, everything that could bear a coat of white paint had it; cellars and darksome corners, usually reserved for the propagation of spiders and evil musty odors, responded wholesomely to the healthful effects of the white-wash brush.[18]

In addition all the backstage personnel — prop men, scene shifters, etc. — were dressed in white coveralls and wore felt slippers while the play was going on. Louisa's mandates were absolute. No one defied them. As Clara Morris noted, "He would have been a rarely reckless actor who had ventured to question the authority of 'The Duchess' in her own bailiwick."[19]

The Arch, like most theatres of the period, was equipped with standard drop-and-wing sets depicting the usual range of possibilities for the typical drama — a parlor, a kitchen, the street, a palace, forest, castles, both interior and exterior, a garden, etc. These were used over and over again.[20] Little attention was paid to the "production values" so dear to the 20th-century theatre. Sets and lights were standard, costumes were up to the actor to provide, and rarely coordinated, and properties and sound effects fell to the hapless stage manager. Nonetheless, standards at the Arch were high and Mrs. Drew exacting. "Mrs. Drew developed a stock company at the Arch Street Theatre that not only was famous throughout the country, but also served as a training school for some of the best actors of later years."[21] Small wonder then that William Winter, then a fledgling critic, was fawningly obsequious when he encountered the Duchess in New York. Her company was, quite simply, the best.

The nucleus of the company did not change greatly from season to season, but, from the beginning, she booked in stars to appear with them, including Edwin Forrest, Edwin Booth, Charlotte Cushman, Joseph Jefferson III, Fanny Davenport, and even John Wilkes Booth in 1863, two years before he was to assassinate President Abraham Lincoln.

When Mrs. Drew began her career as a manager, she performed in 42 plays the first season, and, by her own admission, borrowed money every week to meet the payroll. With experience her expertise grew and though she still borrowed money regularly, she was confident enough to refurbish the theatre, hire more actors and strengthen the season.

However, it was not until John Drew returned from his protracted tour that the theatre finished a season profitably. Drew appeared at the Arch for 100 nights, playing to great acclaim. He performed all the proven hits in his repertoire: Goldfinch in *The Road to Ruin*, O'Bryan in *The Irish Emigrant* and Meddle in *London Assurance* among others. Perhaps it was the least he could do for a wife who genuinely appeared to *believe* that Georgiana's baby was the product of a failed marriage and runaway husband. At any rate the prodigals had been welcomed home, housed, fed and promptly put to work on the Arch Street stage.

Drew's performances were his last, for, in a freak accident, as he was preparing to go to an audition in New York, he tripped on the stair. He was carrying the baby and, in attempting to protect it, struck his own head. The result was an inflammation of the brain from which he never recovered. Mrs. Drew mourned him with genuine fervor and 35 years later wrote of him:

> I don't think there are many persons surviving him now who remember him well, and he was worth remembering; one of the best actors I ever saw, in a long list of the most varied description. Had he lived to be forty-five, he would have been a great actor. But too early a success was his ruin; it left him with nothing to do. Why should he study when he was assured on all sides (except my own) that he was as near perfection as it was possible for man to be? So he finished his brief and brilliant career at thirty-four years of age, about the age when men generally study most steadily and aspire most ambitiously.[22]

Her love was obviously tempered by a clear-eyed view of his faults as well as his virtues.

After his death, the Arch Street Theatre began a period of prosperity under his widow's management. The mortgage and accumulated debts were paid off and the stockholders' shares increased in value. The number and quality of the actors continued to improve, and her repertory became increasingly substantial:

> During the eight-year period of 1861–69 Mrs. Drew managed the Arch Street with a brilliance that has rarely been matched and probably *never* by a woman. She had an eye for talent and knew how to develop it.... Her stock company was not only talented—it was extraordinarily well

> disciplined. And her theatre was more than a theatre. It was a school for
> good manners.[23]

"There was constant variety, constant change and those who were permanent members of the Drew Stock Company were trained in a system of exacting, but invigorating methods,"[24] added Moutrose Moses.

The success of the Arch was undeniable on financial as well as artistic
terms. Box office prices were low when compared with the costs of running
a theatre whose rent alone was $6200 per year. The prices ranged from a
high of 50 cents for the Parquette through 37½ cents for the Dress Circle
and a quarter for the Family Circle to just 15 cents for the Amphitheatre.

Furthermore, Mrs. Drew was at the height of her powers as an actress.
A contemporary described her abilities:

> Mrs. Drew is one of the few instances of a prodigy in youth becoming
> a star in the dramatic constellation. Her greatness does not arise from that
> of the character, but consists in her manner of portraying it. In form,
> stature, mobility of countenance and physique, she is made to give the
> dramatic world assurance of an actress; while a lofty intellect, a pas-
> sionate devotion to her art, and a highly cultivated mind, have stamped
> the seal of excellence on her brow.
>
> Her reading is faultless; her voice is clear, of great compass and musical
> in tone, her enunciation so clear and distinct that you lose no word or
> syllable of the text in her most impassioned utterance. She does not
> "mouth" or "saw the air" as some of our players do, not "tear a passion to
> tatters"; nor does she "o'er step the modesty of nature."
>
> There is a refreshing originality about her conceptions; while to a
> remarkable degree she possesses the talent that makes a bodiless creation
> of the dramatist's mind a living fact, suffused and impregnated with
> natural emotions and desires. It is in the higher range of dramatic acting
> that this lady shines. She invests her characters with a charm that had
> its birth in nature. She disdains the idea of playing to an audience,
> and appealing to its sympathies through the garb only of the character
> in which she appears. In energy, in earnestness of purpose, in fidelity to
> all those minute details delineation which make it perfect, she is the queen
> of her art. She has always possessed a wonderfully quick study, and I am
> told by old actors, who have been members of her company at the "Arch"
> that she was never known to come to even the first rehearsal with the
> book of the play. Whenever a new piece was to be produced, it was first
> read to the company, then rehearsals called. She was always letter
> perfect.[25]

During the period from 1862 to 1880, the Arch Street Theatre and Mrs.
John Drew enjoyed an unprecedented period of prosperity and a number
of actors began their training under her stern but forgiving eye.

> She was always a wonderful disciplinarian; hers was said to be the last of
> those green-rooms that used to be considered schools of good manners.
> Some women descend to bullying to maintain their authority — not so
> Mrs. John Drew. Her armor was a certain chill austerity of manner, her

weapon sharp sarcasm, while her strength lay in her self-control, her self-respect.[26]

Her daughter Georgie, an irrepressible minx, phrased her description of her mother differently, but the picture conjured up is a vivid one. "I distinctly remember the icy politeness in my mother's tone as she would turn to me at rehearsal, when I was gossiping away in a corner instead of attending to my cue, and remark: 'Now, Miss Drew, if you are *quite* ready, we will resume.'"[27]

Like Laura Keene before her, Louisa Lane Drew was known at home and at the theatre as "The Duchess." Georgie remarked, "I suppose it is appropriate enough, but who then could possibly be Queen?"[28]

Among the actors who began careers with the Arch Street Theatre Company were Ada Rehan,[29] Georgie's particular friend; Clara Morris, who was to write a vivid portrait of her mentor, Fanny Davenport; Louis James, who became a crony of Maurice Barrymore; and Stuart Robson. Small wonder that young actors and actresses were awed by association with the Duchess. Her own family was frequently overwhelmed: "the magnitude of my grandmother most struck me. Her power seemed to exude from her regal presence; she was commanding. . . . When, in later years I encountered royalty, nothing surprised me. I had known my grandmother."[30]

The Arch Street company included Frank Murdock, Lizzie Price, wife of writer Charles Fechter, and John Drew's brother Frank, and remained relatively stable from year to year. However, Mrs. Drew had to resort with increasing frequency to employing stars to appear in a single production. Among the notables who played under her aegis were Edwin Booth, Helena Modjeska, J.W. Wallack, Jr., E.L. Davenport, Lotta Crabtree, F.F. MacKay, and Charlotte Cushman.

Eventually these measures proved insufficient to maintain the Arch's repertory stock company, and in 1877 she made the theatre into a combination house. Having been dragged into the new order of theatrical life, she made an abrupt about-face and formed a combination company of her own with Joseph Jefferson.

Jefferson was an old friend and she had known his family all her life, performing as a child with his grandfather. Jefferson had been looking for a property to follow up his successes with the *Rip Van Winkle* tour, and decided to revise *The Rivals* to suit his purposes. Maurice Barrymore frequently joked that Sheridan wouldn't have recognized the script, but Jefferson was a shrewd businessman as well as a fine actor and he knew precisely what his fans wanted his character to be like. He elected to play Bob Acres, a rustic who generates much of the comedy; Mrs. Drew played Mrs. Malaprop. Jefferson admired her work greatly.

> Mrs. Drew . . . introduced some novel business in her first scene with Captain Absolute that struck me as one of the finest points I had ever seen made. When Mrs. Malaprop hands the letter for the Captain to read, by accident she gives him her own love-letter lately received by her from Lucius O'Trigger. As the Captain reads the first line which betrays the secret, Mrs. Drew starts, blushes, and simperingly explains that "there is a slight mistake." Her manner during this situation was the perfection of comedy.[31]

They toured every season for the next 12 years and covered 27,000 miles.

While she was able to keep the Arch's stock company intact, it was recognized as a prime source of new talent for the New York producers. Augustin Daly, emerging as a major figure in the theatre, was a staunch admirer of the Drew company and made frequent visits to scout the Arch for young talented actors to join his Fifth Avenue Theatre. One, so selected, was Louisa's 21-year-old son.

John Drew, Jr., had made his debut with his mother's company at 19 in a small part, Mr. Plumper, as a member of the cast of *Cool as a Cucumber* for his sister's benefit. His mother appeared as the maid in order to ease him through any stagefright. She needn't have bothered. Young Jack was more than equal to the occasion, displaying far too much self-assurance. Mrs. John Drew turned to the audience and shook her head slowly. "What a dreadful young man," she ad libbed. "I wonder what he will be like when he grows up?"[32] Most of the audience, in on the joke, applauded uproariously. Suitably chastened, Jack gave up selling clocks at Wanamaker's, a large Philadelphia department store, and turned to the stage, joining first the Arch company and later Daly's Fifth Avenue. In New York he was not an immediate success, and Daly nearly despaired of young Drew's talents. He gave him one last opportunity, the role of Bob Ruggles in *The Big Bonanza*. This time Jack achieved the lasting success expected of one of his blood. Drew continued to improve as a performer until he became a star at the turn of the century. Moreover, he was blessed with the famous "Drew memory":

> John . . . got back to the Ninth Street house in Philadelphia dog-tired and dispirited after a largely profitless tour with *Diplomacy* at two o'clock on a winter morning. John's mother opened the door to . . . knocking, a candle in one hand and in the other, the script of the old English comedy *Wives as They Were and Maids as They Are* by Mrs. Inchbald. "Don't go to bed, John," commanded that redoubtable woman, handing him the script. "You play this tonight." His role, Mr. Bronzeley, was an exceptionally long one, but by dint of studying it for eight hours without so much as a catnap and attending ten a.m. rehearsal, he sailed through the night's performance letter-perfect.[33]

One of the reasons that Drew performed so poorly at first was simply his eagerness to experience all the delights available in New York City. His companion in these explorations was Maurice Barrymore, son of British pukka sahibs, who had decided to give acting a "go."

Drew brought "Barry" home and his sister Georgie promptly fell in love. Georgie was the beauty of the family, and the full heir to her father's Irish charm and wit as well. She began her career at 16 at the Arch, over her mother's rather feeble protests, and was an immediate audience favorite. Her specialty was light comedy and by the time Barry came calling, she was on her way to stardom.

Maurice Barrymore was charming and Georgie was entranced. Mrs. Drew was less smitten, but unable to deny her favorite daughter her heart's desire. Although Georgie complained about her mother's old-fashioned notions of courtship ("Mother sat at the other end of the drawing room, 'snowing' on us"),[34] young love triumphed and the couple was married on New Year's Eve in 1876. Three children resulted; Lionel, born April 28, 1878, Ethel, August 15, 1879, and Mrs. Drew's favorite, John, born February 14, 1882. All were born at home in Philadelphia under their grandmother's vigilant supervision.

By the time Georgie fell seriously ill, the Arch Street Theatre was facing rough financial waters, and only 14-year-old Ethel could be spared to accompany her consumptive mother West. Three months later she returned with Georgie's body. Within the year, the entire family faced even greater upheaval.

Business had grown increasingly sporadic at the Arch. Despite her decision to replace the repertory with combination companies, Mrs. Drew was never able to wring the same income from the theatre that she had in palmier days. One of her business managers proved to be lining his own pockets at her expense, and in 1892, when she returned from her last Jefferson tour, matters reached an impasse. With great reluctance, she informed the board of directors of the Arch that she was relinquishing the lease of the theatre. It was the end of a 30-year relationship. It was also the end of an era.

Typically, she was reluctant to garner publicity by announcing her departure, and few in the audience of *The Love Chase* knew that as Widow Green, Louisa Lane Drew was appearing for the last time on the Arch Street stage. She toured briefly under her son Sidney's management, but when that too seemed doomed to end in failure, she retreated to New York, to her son John's apartment. Ethel Barrymore came with her:

> Mummum was still there, very reticent, a person of absolutely enormous dignity and silences. She had a comfortable room and she was Mrs. John Drew, Uncle Jack's mother. But is was Uncle Jack's apartment, not her house.... Mummum was unhappy at being dependent for the first time in her life, although it was on her own son, and she was bewildered

... all very tragic for her because she had been such a commanding person with everyone's life in her hands for so many years. But instead of drooping, her back seemed to get straighter and straighter as she gazed out over the sinister rooftops of New York.[35]

However, she retained her powers to the end, and in 1896 she joined an "all-star" cast of *The Rivals*, teaming once more with Joseph Jefferson on the tour. Her vigor was undiminished and her comic sense as strong as ever. The tour played a series of one-night stands on the order of 27 cities in 27 days, and Louisa Lane Drew, reared in the theatre and 76 years old, never once complained.

The following January, she attempted her last role in *The Sporting Duchess*, "the great Drury Lane Melo-Drama," but was forced to withdraw from the cast after only a few performances. The child who blithely sailed through six and seven characters in a single evening had become the old woman who couldn't manage the costume changes.

She took up residence at Bevan House, a boardinghouse in Larchmont. In the summer, her 15-year-old grandson John Barrymore came to keep her company. Their rooms were on the top floor of the house because these were the cheapest, and her legs were failing her so they would make the journey downstairs just once a day in the morning. All day long she would sit on the porch, pretending to read one of the innumerable blue-covered paperback books she brought with her, and remembering old times, old friends, old theatres. Occasionally she would tell John stories, breaking into reminiscences that made little sense to the boy. Once when Lionel visited, he spoke with her doctor and repeated the medic's gloomy diagnosis. She rejected it categorically: "The typical nonsense of his deplorable trade. There is nothing the matter with me at all. I am merely resting between plays. And I must be up soon for a new rehearsal."[36] For once, Louisa was unable to order matters to suit her. Ethel visited briefly from London, with news of her coming season with Sir Henry Irving. When she left, Mrs. Drew was still rocking and reading on the porch, but by the end of the summer she was bedridden and required a nurse in attendance. John remained in Larchmont. On the morning of August 31, she spoke with him at length, and then around noon fell into a light sleep. He left her in the care of the nurse and slipped outside for a few hours. When he returned she had slipped into a coma and newsmen were gathering on the lawn. As if she had been waiting for his return, she had a final convulsion. John saw her die.

Hannah Drew, the elder John Drew's sister, stepped in to prevent the boy from having to deal with funeral arrangements. Louisa Lane Hunt Mossop Drew was buried in the Glenwood Cemetery in Philadelphia. As she had wished, her son had her tombstone inscribed with the following verse:

Life! we've been long together
Through pleasant and through cloudy weather
'Tis hard to part when friends are dear
Perhaps 'twill cause a sigh, a tear;
Then steal away, give little warning,
    Choose thine own time,
    Say not Good Night, but in some brighter clime
    Bid me Good Morning.

Mrs. Drew achieved many things during her lifetime: acclaim as a performer, plaudits as a manager, immense stature in theatre society, recognition by her peers. She made even greater contributions, fashioning a stock company that embodied the discipline she had learned as a child combined with genuine respect for the actor and his craft. She bridged most of the time span of the American theatre, performing as a child with grizzled veterans of the Hallam company, and training the young actors who would become the stars of the early 20th century. As a manager, she broke free of any stigma against "ladies" in the profession by running her theatre brilliantly, creatively, and artistically. Actors were eager to serve under her and to accept her disciplines since they were assured of respect and payment in return.

Mrs. John Drew died at the age of 77. For 76 of those years she had been a performer; for 30, a manager. The theatre was her life. She knew no other way, craved no other, aspired to no other. For her, the theatre was the most wonderful and desirable life anyone would hope to live. She relished its disciplines and accepted its strictures. In the end, the theatre she had known abandoned her, and she was left to live out her days in regrets and memories. Memories of her family and her unceasing devotion to excellence in the theatre are her true memorial, and we may be sure that she never regretted one year at the Arch, or one performance.

Act IV

THE ACTIVISTS

As a general rule, actresses in the 18th and 19th centuries did not involve themselves in political controversies, nor in popular causes. Those attitudes have changed in our own time when name recognition can be crucial to the success of social or moral issues.

However, two 19th century performers did have tremendous impact — one on the theatre and the other on national political decisions. For Mrs. Fiske, her choices were deliberate and her causes chosen. For Fanny Kemble, her route was more roundabout. The words written in sorrow and anger and published with cold resolve had a far-reaching effect which their author could not anticipate.

In both cases, the situation in which these women found themselves was organic — that is, it grew out of their lives and relationships. Neither conciously picked up the cudgels of the "reformer" for the sake of the reforms, but once caught up in the machinery they had inadvertently set in motion, both were able to master the maelstrom, ride out the storm and effect lasting changes.

Perhaps their greatest legacy was their divorce from the event once the desired object was achieved. Fanny Kemble wished to expose the inequalities of slavery in a very particular place and time which was personal to her. She did not become a stump-hopping, strident-voiced abolitionist who abandoned her career for a cause. She simply made her statement, backed it fully, and went on with her life, feeling the statement strong enough to stand on its own.

Mrs. Fiske, in her crusade against the Syndicate, was involved longer and more intimately and carried her cause to the countryside, but this intimacy was inherent in the nature of the conflict. Once the situation was resolved, she too, left it behind and did not become a tiresome celebrity harking back to a moment of triumph. Like Fanny Kemble, she went forward. Both women were apparently unaware of how momentous their influence was to become and how great their impact.

Fanny Kemble

A 19 year old trembled in the wings, swept by waves of stage fright. Lady Capulet summoned her wayward daughter. "Juliet," she called, and with slight hesitation the slim girl put a tentative foot to the stage. Her Aunt Dall gave her a push and as she rushed to the embrace of her stage-mother, the theatre exploded in a roar of welcome. Almost nothing of the first scene could be heard by the enthusiastic crowd gathered to watch the debut of Fanny Kemble, heir to a hundred years of theatrical tradition.

With each passing line, her confidence grew, and with it, her assurance. By the balcony scene, her initial tremors had dissolved as she immersed herself in the role — a young girl, a novice to the stage, experiencing the passions of the adolescent Juliet for the first time, sweeping her audience with her, inviting them to *believe* in the tragedy unfolding before them as *she* believed in the role she was playing.

The audience had been attracted by several advertised novelties. Charles Kemble, a still-dashing matinee idol, was abandoning lovelorn Romeo to play bold, bad Mercutio. His wife, Marie-Therese deCamp, was making an unlikely comeback as Lady Capulet, and their daughter Fanny was beginning her career as a breathtakingly lovely, totally inexperienced Juliet.

The theatergoers, alive to every nuance, found much to adore in Charles' daughter, and by the time of her last tragic scene, they too, wept at the senseless deaths of the young lovers. It was a debut without compare. Cold Londoners took the newcomer to their hearts and thronged the theatre, knowledgeably discussing the skill of the actress and the heritage of her talent. No one, least of all the Kembles, seemed to doubt that her success would continue.

Placing so green an actress on the stage was a move bred of desperation and financial calamity. The Covent Garden Theatre had been the home of the Kemble fortunes, virtually since Roger Kemble's children learned to count a house. It was like a Saint Bernard — familiar, enormous, and hellishly expensive to maintain. Combined with Charles' usual improvident ways and casual (at best) financial planning, it was small wonder that the theatre in which Fanny made her debut was plastered with debtors' notices and tax bills, and in imminent danger of being auctioned to satisfy the more importunate of Charles' creditors.

The Kembles had not always had the succubus of a theatre to account for their ill-fortune. Roger, the "founder" of the dynasty, had pretensions to genteel connections, but like his father, was only an itinerant barber or hairdresser. Bewitched by the players whom he met on the road, he abandoned his razors and strops for an even more uncertain life as a "stroller," an unlicensed actor, drifting from town to town performing hoary old chestnuts for audiences equally composed of country merchants and their servants, and frequently leaving behind props in his haste to avoid capture by the local constabulary.

Along the way Roger acquired a wife, Sarah Ward, 13 children, and some skill at his profession. Most of his children began to perform as soon as they could cross a stage without falling off it, and several of them became the leading actors of their day.

Roger, true to his genteel pretensions, found the money to send the boys to a Catholic school near Douai, and the girls to a governess. He sternly forbade their adult interest in the stage. If he intended to fire their theatrical desires, he could hardly have chosen a more effective means. Sarah Kemble, his daughter, was the first to disobey. She married another stroller, Henry (Tom) Siddons, almost certainly to disoblige her father, and then began to perform as Mrs. Sarah Siddons. In time she became the greatest tragedienne of the century. Totally devoid of a sense of humor, she was "the Complete Tragic Muse" off-stage as well as on, and often lapsed into blank verse while ordering her breakfast chocolate. Today, her name is still a touchstone for the more intense styles of acting.

Her brother, John Philip, abandoned his father's priestly plans for him, and followed Sarah on to the stage, playing tragic heroes given to bombast and much sword-play. Soon the name "Kemble" became synonymous with the finest acting of the age, and at least five other Kemble brothers and sisters took to the stage. Some were reasonably successful, others less so, but as its sons and daughters followed them on the boards, the Kemble dynasty dominated English theatre from the mid-1700s to the 1890s. They were justly known as "the most distinguished actor-family England has ever produced."[1]

One sister, Eliza Kemble Whitelock, achieved marked success in America where she was a notable early "leading lady" with a somewhat regrettable reputation. However, the true black sheep of the family was sister Ann, who made a bigamous early marriage and then started her stage career by giving "instructive lectures on sexual habits" illustrated by *live*, scantily clad models in "Temples of Health." John Philp and Sarah eventually made her a miserly allowance and quartered her outside London. Her next appearance was at a bawdy house where she was shot in the face by a recalcitrant customer.[2]

The boys turned out a little better. Stephen became a noted provincial manager and actor. He achieved the kind of staid respectability that allowed his daughter to marry the grandson of wealthy inventor Sir Richard Arkwright.[3] Charles, defying John Philip's paterfamilias edict, went on the stage in his turn, and became the handsome, romantic, second lead the family needed to round out their private casting pool. He fell in love with Marie-Therese deCamp,[4] an enchanting and virtuous young French actress

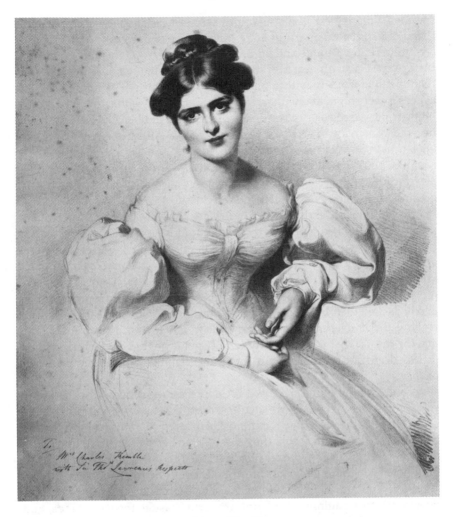

Fanny Kemble

in John Philip's company, but it is remarkable that their marriage ever took place.

John Philip, one of the legendary topers in a century noted for this indulgence, one evening took a drunken notion to ravish the "ravissant" Mlle. deCamp. Her screams brought timely intevention, and John Philip was eventually forced to make a public apology — in print — which assured all that her virtue was unsullied. When she and Charles became involved, John Philip again intervened, proclaiming a *five year* waiting period until Charles' thirtieth birthday. Amazingly Charles agreed to this delay in his wedding plans. Marie-Therese was less meek, and less faithful, but after the specified time period, the couple did wed. Their daughter Frances Anne (Fanny) Kemble was born in 1809, one of five children.

John Philip Kemble and Sarah Siddons undertook the management of the Covent Garden Theatre in 1803. When the unlucky house burned, they rebuilt it handsomely with money loaned by a variety of noblemen. The expenses were high, and with irrefutable logic, the Kembles decided to pass on their increased costs to the ticket-purchasing public. The ensuing fracas became known as the O.P., or Old Price Riots. After two weeks of rioting audiences, cat-calls, fisticuffs, and threats of grievous bodily harm, the Kembles quietly reduced the prices, painted over the damage done to their new façade, and gave up higher ticket prices as a lost cause. The theatre continued to incur ever greater indebtedness.

John Philip's friends eventually forgave the £10,000 they'd loaned, and the Kembles lurched along, performing amid ongoing fiscal panic.

In time Sarah Siddons retired, and John Philip quick-wittedly acquired a £1,000 annuity and retired to Switzerland, *giving* the management of the family white elephant to brother Charles in 1822. It was not a kind act.

Charles was even less thrifty than his elder brother and sister had been, and he lacked their big-name drawing power. The Covent Garden Theatre wallowed ever deeper into a morass of debt, and it was to rescue the family and the theatre that young Fanny Kemble made her bid for theatrical fame. A less desperate manager than her father would never have taken the chance.

Fanny had previously shown little interest in or talent for the family profession. Her girlhood was spent disrupting whatever boarding school she attended whenever her parents remembered to retrieve her from the assorted relations with whom they'd deposited her, while off on tour. From this unusual upbringing, she retained certain interests which were to remain with her throughout her adult life. She adored the poetry of Byron, then considered not quite "nice" reading for a well-brought-up young lady. She developed strong affinities for Edinburgh, the seaside, the woodlands, and, from her mother, a devotion to fishing. Her schooling provided flawless French, meticulous grammar, and no mathematics at all. The military drillmaster at a nearby battlefield encampment helped her achieve a ramrod posture which made the most of her scant height. Conspicuously absent in this catalogue of interests and accomplishments, though, were the elocution lessons, amateur theatricals and walk-ons in small roles, usually endemic to offspring of the theatrical community. Evidently, she did not feel their lack.

As she grew older, Fanny developed an ambition to write, and at 17 began a long historical novel loosely based on the life of Francis I. This transformed itself into a play which was published and later performed. She had begun work on a second drama when the family finances collapsed.

During her respites from literary composition she memorized the role of "Juliet," a task suggested by her mother who was very careful never to suggest that Juliet would make a splendid vehicle for Fanny's theatrical debut. Instead the effort seems to have been regarded as a lesson set-piece, rather as similar young girls, then in convent schools, committed huge chunks of the Bible to memory.

To demonstrate her mastery of this mnemonic feat, Fanny recited the role to her father. Marie-Therese read the cues, and Charles was visibly moved by his daughter's recitation. He took Fanny to Covent Garden to recite from the stage, and, satisfied that her voice had sufficient power, resolved to make a final last-ditch effort to recoup his debts by introducing this incandescent new Juliet. Charles may have been a charming womanizer, a second rate actor, and an insatiable drinker like his brother, but he possessed shrewd theatrical instincts.

Three frantic weeks of rehearsal followed. The cast drew from the entire family. Charles played Mercutio, Marie-Therese took Lady Capulet. Marie's sister Adelaide oversaw the costumes, and Sarah Siddons coached the young actress. Henry, Fanny's 15-year old brother, was auditioned for Romeo, but he was histrionically hopeless, and in fact, never acted. William Abbott was finally selected to play the lovestruck youth.

After his daughter's sensational debut on October 5, 1829, Charles built a season around Fanny and was able to keep the theatre out of the red for a time and pay back, or have forgiven, most of Covent Garden's debts. London flocked to see his talented daughter play Juliet, and later most of Shakespeare's other heroines. For her part, Fanny was excited about the £30 a week *she* was making and promptly began to take riding lessons.

However, by far the most important result of her new-found theatrical fame had nothing to do with saving the theatre or paying debts. A craze for Fanny Kemble had swept London and anything that astounding young woman could produce was readily snapped up. Sophisticated Londoners were astonished to discover that the lovely young actress was a playwright as well. They clamored to read the drama she'd produced. As each edition of her play sold out to an adoring public, her publishers brought out another, so her success was both theatrical and literary. She basked in this limelight as only a 19-year old celebrity can. For two and a half years, she was the darling of London.

In 1832, she and Charles embarked on a major and very lucrative tour of America. For all her seeming sophistication, Fanny had never been to the country before, and she found herself entranced by the welcome she received. To be sure America had far fewer people than England and far fewer amenities, but the entire country seemed to rise up and embrace the new English star!

Fanny was lionized and adored. She played to enthusiastic, sold-out audiences. Joseph Ireland records an account of her American triumphs:

> [A]ll hearts and hands were eager to give her a cordial welcome. Her
> triumph here was complete; she was the acknowledged Queen of Tragedy
> from Boston to New Orleans, without a rival near her throne.... No ac-
> tress that preceded her in America ever held so powerful and deep a sway
> over the hearts and feelings of her auditors.[5]

The critics were no less unanimous in their praise. Representative of
his fellows is the reviewer for the *New York Mirror*. "Miss Fanny Kemble
did not disappoint expectations. Of higher praise she cannot be ambitious
for never was expectation raised to such a pitch.... Her acting is most easy
and elegant ... and perfectly original in our eyes ... [no other actress]
could ... exceed ... the grace and deep power of Fanny Kemble."[6] She and
Charles had never been so well-received nor so highly paid in London, and
the leading hostesses of New York, Philadelphia and Boston vied to entertain the Kembles.

One such party was to change her life forever. She was introduced to
Pierce Butler, the handsome, elegant grandson of a Georgia planter. Pierce
loved horses and so did Fanny. She loved the water; his plantation was surrounded by it. These and other common likes drew them together. Soon
flirtation had given way to courtship, and as the courtship grew ever deeper
and more intense, Fanny found herself being swept off her feet.

The man who had captured her heart was the scion of a wealthy
American family. His grandfather, the original Pierce Butler, was an
English soldier who had cast his lot with the colonists in the Revolution and
married the daughter of a South Carolina planter. One of his four
daughters, Sarah, married a Philadelphia physician named Mease. When
her father died, he left his plantation jointly to his unwed daughter Frances,
and to Sarah's boys, John and Butler, with the proviso that to inherit, they
had to assume the surname of Butler. Butler legally changed his name to
Pierce Mease Butler. Later John, too, adopted his grandfather's name. The
Butler family was essentially Philadelphian with a source of income from
the South. For most of the year, they were absentee landlords who
sometimes spent the worst of the winter months visiting Georgia, but they
were primarily content to leave the day-to-day running of the plantation
to managers. Pierce, Fanny's fiancé was no different from his relations. His
upbringing had been that of a young gentleman of leisure and wealth, entitled to his place in society, and as far as he was concerned, his home was
a mansion in Philadelphia at the corner of Eighth and Spruce. By nature
Pierce was amiable, vacillating, and attractive. All the qualities which first
attracted Fanny to him — his manners, his studied affectations of culture
and indolence, his generosity, and his deft way with women — were later
to prove to be her chief complaints against him. His virtues had become
faults when magnified by the glare of incompatibility.

When Pierce proposed, she cast her fledgling career to the winds and enthusiastically embraced the idea of becoming the pampered, adored wife of a plantation owner. Charles was hardly so enthusiastic, but in the face of Fanny's ardent pleas, he could scarcely prevent the marriage. Neither of them knew what she had let them in for.

After the wedding on June 20, 1834, Fanny and Pierce settled into life in the Butler home. Fanny was only too willing to abandon the stage, and she gave a farewell performance two weeks after her wedding. The couple had two children, daughters Frances (Fan) and Sarah (Sally), and the first years of their married life were marred only by Fanny's increasing awareness of the plight of the American slave population. During her performances, she had become acquainted with the Sedgwick family and William Ellery Channing. These people were among the literate elite of New England, and they also held strong antislavery views. Fanny was naturally sympathetic to them, given her English upbringing, and embraced the less radical aspects of their philosophy wholeheartedly. Pierce was appalled, and their family discussions began to grow increasingly acrimonious. To her Butler relations, she was regarded as little better than an abolitionist, and Pierce's folly in marrying a "play-actress" was reinforced.

When Frances Butler, Pierce's aunt, died, matters came to a head. Despite his brother John's protests, Pierce reluctantly agreed to take his wife and family South with him when he went to Georgia to settle the estate, and claim his share of the plantation. Fanny was eager to experience firsthand the evils of slavery and to convert Pierce to her way of thinking. She also intended to write a personal account of plantation life. Her inspiration was a journal kept by English playwright and author Matthew Gregory Lewis who had inherited a West Indies sugar plantation and then recorded the conditions there upon his visit. She intended that her account would be "free from misstatements, or rather, misstakes"[7] and contain only "details . . . which come under my immediate observations."[8] If Pierce had known the troubles that would have arisen out of this single trip South, he would have dissuaded Fanny from accompanying him, or if that proved impossible, prevented her from any access to paper and ink during her stay there. The world would have been poorer for such a loss.

Pierce, Fanny and the girls traveled South together. It was December. Grimly Fanny tried to enjoy the rough corduroy roads, and the warmth, and to deny the queasiness she felt from riding all day in an enclosed coach. The journey from Philadelphia to Georgia took nine days. Little did she realize that the truly horrible part of the experience lay ahead.

Butler's plantation was huge and very isolated. She felt stranded, alien, isolated, abruptly cut off from the life she had known. She was bewildered as well by a totally foreign lifestyle. The girl who had run wild much of her life, found herself a virtual prisoner with her every movement prescribed. By the time she'd lived at the plantation for several months, she fully understood the nature of the plantation economy, and it disturbed her immeasurably.

The academic descriptions of slavery which had so revolted her in abolitionist tracts and which she had wanted to see in person were far more disgusting than she expected. The house servants who had been selected to wait on them were "perfectly filthy in their persons and their clothes — their faces, hands and naked feet being liberally encrusted with dirt . . ."[9] Fanny found it easier to dispense with their presence than to endure it during meals. No doubt, she was considered very strange. Her maid, Mary, also, distressed her. "Mary . . . is so intolerably offensive in her person that it is impossible to endure her proximity."[10] Despite these experiences, Fanny refused to accept the usual Southern argument, that the smell and dirt were inherent with the "Negro race" and therefore a reason to keep them enslaved. Instead she declared, "I cannot imagine that they would smell much worse if they were free"[11], and "I . . . believed that peculiar ignorance of the laws of health and the habits of decent cleanliness are the real and only causes of this disagreeable characteristic of the race."[12]

Fanny carried her investigations of the conditions of Mr. Butler's slaves further and discovered that they were allowed only two meals daily and the first of these could not be eaten until they had been in the fields for several hours. Their other meal they took after the day's work was finished. Furthermore, they were denied most of the amenities, "Chairs, tables, plates, knives, forks, they had none; they sat . . . on the earth or doorsteps, and ate, either out of their little cedar tubs or an iron pot, some few with broken iron spoons, more with pieces of wood, and all the children with their fingers."[13]

Fanny began to oversee the infirmary, which appalled her:

> [T]hese last poor wretches lay prostrate upon the floor, without bed, mattress, or pillow, buried in tattered and filthy blankets, which huddled round them as they lay strewed about, left hardly space to move upon the floor. . . . Here lay some burning with fever, others chilled with cold and aching with rheumatism . . . and dirt, noise and stench, and every aggravation of which sickness is capable . . . here they lay like brute beasts. . . .[14]

She plunged into introducing more hygenic conditions, but it was an uphill battle, understood by neither the whites nor the blacks.

She also made an effort to induce the slaves to clean their huts which were "filthy, cold, and wretched"[15] by "bidding [them] kindle up the fire, sweep the floor, and expel the poultry."[16] She met with little success. "For a long time my very words seemed unintelligible to them"[17] and despite demonstrations of her meaning, she made little impact on the lifestyle of the Butler slaves.

She begged Pierce to free his slaves. Gently he explained that that was not possible. The arguments increased and grew more shrill and harsh. Fanny demanded, Pierce denied. Fanny ordered, Pierce refused. Fanny sobbed, Pierce stood resolute. It quickly became known the length and breadth of the plantation that Butler's bride was little better than an abolitionist! Soon the couple was arguing about everything—money, their children, Fanny's desire to return to the stage, politics, and slavery, always slavery. Their marriage began to disintegrate.

As she had when she was a girl, Fanny turned to her pen to express her true feelings. Into her journal she poured every episode of injustice to the slaves, every cruel act, every instance that aroused her ire. Later this journal would become a powerful tool in the hands of English and American abolitionists. The conditions which surrounded her were too appalling, the lifestyle too dispiriting, to be borne, without in some way dissipating their effects on her nervous system.

In April of 1839, they left Butler's Island, and returned to the North. Fanny was leaving behind the disgusting conditions on which she'd had so little impact, but she carried with her the journal and strong antislavery views.

In Philadelphia, the arguments continued. Almost daily Pierce explained to her that the very food her children ate and the clothing she wore were dependent upon continuing the system of slavery. However, economics were a poor argument to a woman who had earned a small fortune by performing on the stage, and blithely signed it over to her improvident papa.

Fanny had begun to long for the stage again. The profession she had laid aside so casually beckoned now like a siren's torch. The drudgery of rehearsals and nightly performances seemed a paradise compared to the infamy with which she had been surrounded and which she had discovered herself powerless to change.

Finally her spirit revolted and she fled. In doing so, she left behind her children and her girlhood, and embarked on the long arduous path to regain her fame. She wrote to Pierce,

> I have determined . . . I will no longer be dependent upon you. . . . I can no longer rely upon you. My comfort and happiness, are, as you say, your business, but, as like most of your business, you neglect them utterly. I will so far see to them myself that I will no longer submit to live upon your relations . . . I can obtain . . . for myself, a home, no matter how poor. . . . I will live thus no longer. . ."[18]

When Pierce's importunities proved useless, they entered upon a long and distressing period of divorce proceedings. Pierce Butler replied,

> On my soul and conscience, I have done everything in my power to make you happy. . . . The fault has been entirely your own. . . . If you will govern your irritable temper, and if you can consent to submit your will

to mine, we may be reconciled and happy. I firmly believe that husband and wife cannot live together happily upon any other terms.[19]

Their differences were first a matter of a separation. The Butlers reconciled periodically, mostly "for the children," once spending two and a half years in London where Pierce learned for the first time, the social advantages of a well-connected, if theatrical, wife. The homes of Fanny's friends made his American mansion look paltry.

The ongoing battles between them raged. He constantly reminded her of wifely duties as seen from the perspective of a husband of the 1800s. Fanny riposted with his bad financial management and sexual peccadilloes (slaves in Georgia, housemaids in London), which a *proper* wife of the period would *never* have been able to mention (the humiliation would have been too great). Fanny not only mentioned it, she threw it in Butler's face, along with demands for a substantial allowance, separate accommodations within the same home, and equal access to their children. A modern judge would be only too familiar with these requests, but Pierce had never encounted anything like them. Periodically she would run away, pack her bags and storm off in all directions. Butler was always able to bring her to heel by threatening to remove the children. Adding to Fanny's discontent were two factors: She continued to be totally dependent, financially, on her husband — not at all unusual for the time, but intolerable to a woman who had tasted the joys of independence with her stage earnings.

Secondly, her sister Adelaide, having studied for many years, was making a splash as an exciting new opera star. Like Fanny, many years before, her performances were rescuing Covent Garden from threatened ruin under Charles' management. Fanny was proud of her sister, but she had been off the stage for ten years and the kudos Adelaide was garnering must have been bittersweet. During the time in London, Fanny published excerpts from her journal of her journey South. Pierce was furious and humiliated, and when an abolitionist heard of the diary and approached Fanny to include her views of slavery in a pamphlet, she had to refuse. Pierce absolutely forbade it.

The Butlers were still nominally a family when they returned to America. Pierce ensconced them in an upper class boardinghouse, while renting his own home, which Fanny found degrading. She reacted childishly and once more their marriage began to disintegrate, this time forever. She threatened to return to her career on the stage — a resource denied most young 19th-century wives. Pierce refused to countenance "the public display of his children's mother."

By 1845, she was allowed only an hour a day with the girls. Other access was smugly denied by their English governess whose relationship with Butler was suspect. That summer, Sally and Fan were completely removed from contact with their mother, and it would be five years before she saw them again.

Fanny returned to England, 36, a failed wife, penniless, and dependent. Her life was a shambles. The children were denied to her. She had no income unless she returned to the stage which was certain to precipitate a divorce. Her life had become a textbook display of the old adage, "Marry in haste, repent in leisure."

Following a year in Italy to recuperate and recover from the emotional wrenches she had suffered, Fanny returned to the stage. London managers were uninterested, so she embarked on a provincial tour, stouter, out of practice, and out of fashion. Her performances did attract a certain audience out of curiosity.

To be sure, her performances had a novelty about them that most other performers in the company lacked. William Davidge, in his book *Footlight Flashes*, recounts one such incident

> I must . . . credit Mrs. Butler [Fanny Kemble] . . . with introducing a verse of a popular negro melody descriptive of a voyage down the Ohio River in company with a boatman, in the third act of *School For Scandal*.
> The audience were somewhat taken aback by the rendering of the character of Lady Teazle, and stared at each other with mute astonishment and wonder.[20]

The engagement commenced on her return home from America in 1847 at Manchester. She played six nights and "it is to be regretted that the number of visitors to the theatre decreased perceptibly at each representation."[21] Eventually the manager of the Princess Theatre offered her £15 a week (Manchester had paid her £40) and she returned to the London stage. Her costar was William Charles MacReady whose opinion of her abilities was low. She was "ignorant of the first rudiments of her art . . . affected, monotonous, without one real impulse — never in the feeling of the character, never true in look, attitude, or tone. She can never be an actress and this I never ventured to think before."[22] The engagement was not a success. She and MacReady cordially disliked one another and had no respect for the other. Their approach to roles was totally different. MacReady was studious and thorough; Fanny relied on brilliance and inspiration (for which she was chided by her aunt Sarah Siddons). Despite their differences, their careers had many similarities. They had both gone on the stage as teenagers, both in the title roles of *Romeo and Juliet*, both to rescue the family fortunes. Both disliked the theatre and their profession, but MacReady took more personally the onus placed upon unsuccessful actors. Fanny as a Kemble, with their status as a "first family of the theatre," mingled with society and generally escaped the opprobrium heaped on her fellows. MacReady's father had been a regional manager, and he had felt the discrimination against actors keenly when he first came to London.

The battle of wills continued throughout their engagement, and audiences must sometimes have been very puzzled by what they saw.

Unquestionably Fanny lacked stage discipline and was inclined to do exactly as she pleased. This kind of behavious shocked and bewildered MacReady who took his profession very seriously indeed. No doubt it added to the dislike MacReady already felt for his costar. Then, too, Fanny's sentiments were rather "American" and she expressed them freely. MacReady disliked most things "American" so the tension behind their footlights must have been considerable.[23] It served to remind Fanny of everything she most disliked about the theatre and after her contract ended, she withdrew from the stage forever.

She was, of course, still desperately in need of money. Pierce was less than faithful in sending her allowance, and she had just eliminated one of her few lucrative options.

Fanny was left with her pen and her voice. She'd been able to publish an account of her sojourn in Italy, and she began to prepare for publication further reminiscences. In addition, she began a second performance career as a reader. Dramatic readings were something of a family tradition. Mrs. Siddons gave readings of *Macbeth* and Milton, and Charles, Fanny's father, had resumed the custom when he retired as Examiner of Plays. Now he handed over to his daughter the massive volume of Shakespeare passed on from his sister Sarah, from which he habitually read. It was carefully marked with all the cuts and emphases necessary to make a two hour performance from a five act play. Fanny embarked on her new career without a pause. She was delighted never again to have to endure a second rate company and a third rate script. Readings were very popular in Victorian times, and Charles had even been summoned to give them privately for the royal family. Fanny was able to make quite a nice living from them. They attracted a large audience including those whose religious beliefs forbade them from ever setting foot in a theatre.

Henry Austin Clapp, a dramatic critic, paints for us a picture of the success and methods of Fanny Kemble, reader of Shakespeare.

> I listened to her delivery of *The Merry Wives of Windsor,* and was one of an audience which laughed itself almost faint over her interpretation of Falstaff. A middle-aged Englishwoman, in usual afternoon costume, read from an ungarnished platform, out of a big book.... Some thirty years later I was present at Mr. Beerbohm Tree's opening night . . . and saw the leading actor . . . assisted by an accomplished company, using all the appliances of an excellent stage — succeed in carrying the part . . . of Falstaff . . . through an entire evening without once evoking a laugh for his incomparably humorous text.[24]

Fanny was very successful in her readings, and she needed to be for in 1848 Pierce Butler sued for divorce. She had to return to America to appear at the trial. She continued to give her readings in America to pay her living and legal expenses. Once Fanny began to make a little money, she saved it assiduously. One effect of her failed marriage and its consequent financial uncertainties was to make her a hoarder. Unfortunately she had to invest in the name of a spinster friend, for if she'd banked the money under her own name, Pierce and his lawyers could have seized it. No married woman had the right to hold money in her own name in the 1840s.

The divorce proceedings dragged on for a year, marked by Butler's characteristic vacillations and by Fanny's uncertainty that she was doing what was right. Eventually Butler agreed that she might have an income of $1,500 a year, and see the girls for two months every summer if she would let the divorce proceed uncontested with no references to his own misconduct. She acceded to his wishes. The decree was granted in November 1849. Fanny was free of her husband and 40 years old.

Now she began to live life as she chose. She loved the Lenox area in the Berkshires in Massachusetts (what is now Tanglewood) and purchased property there. In time, the natives came to accept the eccentricities of their famous resident. She fished, she wore loose trousers, she rode alone, she didn't water her punch and so got all the "best" inhabitants quite drunk at tea one day, and she read unexpurgated versions of Shakespeare's bawdier plays at public performances:

> Ladies and gentlemen, I have been met in my robing room by a committee . . . and requested not to read *The Merry Wives of Windsor* . . . I have been met in my robing room by the clergymen of your town and they have requested me not to read *The Merry Wives of Windsor*. I have been met in my robing room by a committee of the schoolteachers of your town and they have requested me not to read *The Merry Wives of Windsor*. Ladies and Gentlemen, I shall have the honour of presenting to you this evening Shakespeare's immortal play *The Merry Wives of Windsor*. [25]

A number of proto-feminists and early suffragettes approached her about joining their causes as word of the conditions of her marriage filtered out. (About 18 months after the divorce, Pierce published an ill-considered, but beautifully bound, privately printed, account of his side in the divorce action.) Fanny was enjoying her freedom too greatly to align herself with *any* cause, though her sympathies were clearly with the groups seeking to enlarge the miserably few rights of married women.

She continued to see her daughters for the allotted two months in summer until they turned 21 and were free of the settlement agreement. They remained disconcertingly loyal to Pierce, particularly Frances, and although Fanny deplored the way they had been brought up, she was markedly proud of her "chicks." After the divorce, Pierce didn't fare as well as Fanny. He grew increasingly reckless with money and was caught in the panic of 1857. His slaves had to be sold at auction to satisfy his creditors. It was the largest slave sale that had ever been held in America, netting almost a third of a million dollars. Several years later, when the Civil War broke out, Pierce hinted publicly that he was involved with at least one secret mission back to Georgia with money for the Confederacy. Not surprisingly he was arrested in Philadelphia, and imprisoned for a time, worrying his daughters nearly frantic. Eventually they obtained Lincoln's personal permission to visit him in prison, and then he was released on a kind of personal recognizance. After the war he and Frances returned to the Georgia plantation and ran it for several years, resurrecting as much of its destroyed economy as possible. Frances continued with the plantation after his death, managing it alone for three years until her marriage. One suspects that Fanny was secretly rather proud of her gumption, however much public grumbling there might have been.

Fanny was passionately Unionist and abolitionist in her sentiments. She stayed in America until early 1863 when she was forced to return to England to give a series of the readings, which were no longer profitable in the war-wracked North. She found England in turmoil. Daily the country edged closer to embracing the Confederacy militarily, because of the North's economic embargoes. England's big mills demanded lots of cotton to operate and cotton was rotting on the Southern wharves blockaded by Yankee troops.

For a number of years her *Journal of a Residence on a Georgia Plantation* had circulated privately among her friends in the New England intelligentsia. She had written it with an eye to publication, but her marital difficulties had precluded that possibility. Later when she was free of her husband, she was still reluctant to publish, because she was afraid that it might affect the terms of the settlement and that Pierce might attempt to deny her the visits from her daughters every summer. Now that they were both over 21, the last barrier to her book had fallen. Moreover, she felt that England *needed* to read her book now. Daily the talk of assistance to the Confederacy grew louder and Fanny could see that this might be a death knell for the Unionist cause. She hurried to find a publisher for her diary of life in the South. *Uncle Tom's Cabin* was already telling a fictionalized and dramatized version of slave life. Now she would reveal a nonfiction picture of reality.

By the time the diary was published in May 1863, much of the urgency had dissipated. The South had lost a major battle and the Emancipation Proclamation had altered the political thinking of some in Parliament. Nonetheless, the diary had great impact, perhaps because it made no attempt to varnish the truth. Slaves smelled and had fleas, were brutish and ignorant, and Fanny had disliked some of them and hated their life. The very graphic nature of her picture combined with her personal notoriety got the book before the reading public. Some authorities contend that the American South, during Reconstruction and later, gave the book greater credit than it deserved for its impact on the British[26], but it cannot be denied that Parliament stepped back from the fatal step of a declaration of assistance, or that quotations from *Georgia Plantation* were bandied about in those halls, during the debates. In that moment the defeat of the South was sealed. If the book had been published before *Uncle Tom's Cabin* diluted its impact, there would have been less question regarding its effect. The constraints she felt against early publication may have robbed the book of the benefits it might have derived from being the first, but no one can deny that it was (and is) an impressive statement against the horrors of slavery.

In essence the book was the last remainder of her conscience-stricken girlhood. With its publication she fulfilled all the promises she had made two decades earlier. She could now relax gracefully into late middle age and rejoice in the life she had created for herself out of the shambles of her past.

Fanny gave up the readings in 1869. She was growing stouter, and her voice and hearing were no longer reliable. Her nest egg was substantial and she was well and truly independent — by her own efforts.

She took to publishing her memoirs — *Georgia Plantation* was followed by *Recollections of a Girlhood,* and then by *Recollections of a Later Life* — to the acute distress of her daughter Frances who fretted about the role Pierce might play in her too-candid Mama's accounts of her life. Fanny, as usual, was adamant. She'd print exactly what she chose and that was that.

She spent the last 14 years of her life in England, living part of the time with Frances who had married the clergyman son of a noble British family, the Reverend Canon J. Leigh. Frances returned with him to England after several years of attempts to keep the plantation going. Sarah had married a Philadelphia physician, Dr. Owen Wister. Their namesake son inherited his grandmother's literary aspirations and was the author of *The Virginian,* a classic western novel.

In later years, Fanny became quite close to Henry James, telling him stories of her family and her own exploits which sometimes found themselves transformed by his careful pen. (*Washington Square* is based on an episode in the life of Fanny's reckless brother Henry.[27]) As Fanny aged, she developed eccentricities. She became a "clockwork dresser" who could no more wear Tuesday's evening gown on Thursday, than she could stop wearing wool next to her skin before June 1 whatever the heat. She also became dutiful about her correspondence, frantically answering each letter the day it was received and refusing to write to anyone extempore. She purchased a typewriter, shortly after they were introduced, and was enthusiastic enough about the machine to use one to work on her memoirs (which makes her possibly the first writer to use one).

Towards the end, she did not receive visitors, nor go out, and she was sometimes a trial to her daughter Frances whom she alternately berated and reviled. Always conscious of money, she spent her last years giving it away to the servants, to the distress of her daughters who questioned her competence because of this unaccustomed generosity.

Fanny died in 1893 at the age of 84, and was buried in her father's grave. She was a Kemble through and through, destined for fortune's favor and fame's grace, with enough talent for two professions — actress and author — and with a heedless determination to mold life to her specifications. She compromised badly, and accepted interim defeats with petulance and much temper. She surrounded her life with drama, yet dispised the making of drama upon the stage for a livelihood. She wrote a moving indictment of a social system and contributed to its downfall; and carved a life for herself when propriety dictated that she was "divorced and disgraced." Her eccentricities and enthusiasms were legion, and she behaved as a grand dame might, without any inherited right to the courtesies of nobility.

Fanny Kemble was an original who patterned her existence on an interior plan whose shape only she could perceive. It made her a strong, sometimes notorious, and always interesting person. Her 84 years were not wasted.

Minnie Maddern Fiske

Mrs. Fiske

Staccato, hurried, nervous, brisk,
  Cascading, intermittent, choppy.
The brittle voice of Mrs. Fiske
  Shall serve now as copy.

Time was, when first that voice I heard,
  Despite my close and tense endeavor,
When many an important word
  Was lost and gone forever
Though unlike others at the play,
I never whispered: "Wha'd 'd she say?"

Somewords she runstogetherso;
  Some others are distinctly stated
Somecometoofast and s o m e t o o s l o w
  And some are syncopated,
And yet no voice — I am sincere —
Exists that I prefer to hear.

For what is called "intelligence"
  By every Mrs. Fiskeian critic
As usual is just a sense
      Of humor, analytic.
So anytime, I'm glad to frisk
Two bones to witness Mrs. Fiske.

FPA[1]

Like Franklin P. Adams, audiences had been gladly coming to see Minnie Maddern Fiske most of her life. When she was three she made her first recorded appearance as the Duke of York in *Richard III*, and from then on, played the standard repertoire of roles for juvenile actors ranging from Little Eva in *Uncle Tom's Cabin*, to Mary Morgan in *Ten Nights in a Barroom* and Prince Arthur in *King John*. She played Willie Lee in *Hunted Down* for Laura Keene who was so taken with her that in one of her famous enthusiasms, Miss Keene asked for and got permission to take her on tour as a companion. Minnie was six. Laura Keene was notoriously fickle and when Carlotta Leclerq "borrowed" little Minnie Maddern for *A Wolf in Sheep's Clothing* and advertised it as "her first appearance on any stage," Miss Keene's interest waned. Perhaps she blamed the child for this patent falsehood. At any rate Little Minnie Maddern was that rarity — a child star who passed seamlessly into adult stardom with no awkward ages in between. She came from a theatrical tradition, and knew the stage with all its faults as well as anyone.

Her grandmother was an aristocratic hoyden who ran away with her music master. Conventionally, she was cut off without a shilling and left to starve. Instead she and her husband produced seven musical offspring and sailed to America where they formed the famous Maddern Family Band, and toured as a novelty musical act. Later, the three girls, Elizabeth, Mary and Emma, were the Singing Maddern Sisters. Mrs. Maddern was a strong-willed, theatrical matriarch who looked after her girls and their reputations. She was reluctant to let Lizzie marry Tom Davey, a stagestruck Welsh farmboy turned stage manager on whom she'd set her heart, but the girl was determined and eventually the pair was wed. The marriage was never a success. Tom was improvident and never able to escape his domineering mother-in-law who seemed to cast an evil eye on all his doings. One day he went off on tour to the West and never returned. Before he left, however, he and Lizzie produced their only offspring, Mary Augusta Davey, known professionally as Little Minnie Maddern, then Minnie Maddern, and finally as Mrs. Fiske. She was born in New Orleans in 1865.

When Minnie was touring some years later as a hardened ten-year-old professional, she was somewhat taken aback to be enthusiastically embraced by a short, red-haired, theatre manager in Detroit.

"Minnie, honey, I'm your father," he explained hastily. "Don't you remember me?"

Davey had remarried and fathered a second family and was living in Canada, commuting daily to his American theatre. He died the following year.

Minnie adored her mother who was quite lovely. Occasionally Lizzie would go off on tour and leave Minnie with her mother or sisters. Once the

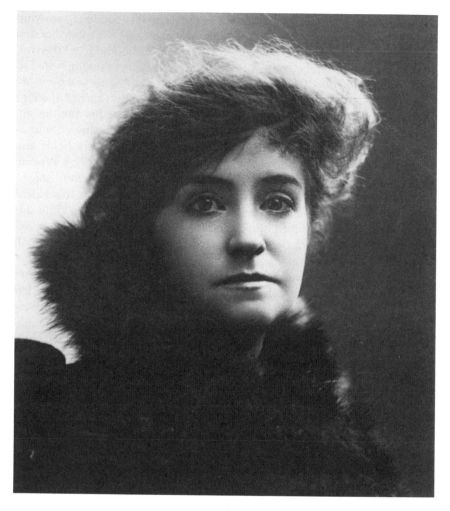

Minnie Maddern Fiske

child was old enough to realize what was happening, she was old enough to protest — vociferously. Even the addition to the household of a new puppy was not enough to quiet her screams for her mother. Finally, exasperated and worn out, her grandmother dumped her on a train and sent her off to Pittsburgh. She arrived there, not knowing where her mother was staying and with only the sketchiest of other information. But she knew quite well who the manager of the company was — after all, she'd appeared for him before — and assumed that he would be staying in the best hotel in town, so that's were she told the hack to take her. Her surmise was correct and she woke him at an ungodly hour, demanding to be taken to her mother.

Eight year old Minnie joined the tour *with* her puppy. It seems probable that Lizzie was less than delighted, but after that she kept the litle girl with her. Lizzie's engagements took them to New York and points east and west. From the time she was ten, Minnie was a useful utility woman in the company, playing any and all roles including boys and old women. She was twelve when she stepped in as the Widow Melnotte in *The Lady of Lyons* when the "old woman" was taken ill. By then she was adept at the professional side of the theatre, and no longer had to be bribed with lollipops to learn her lines as old Barry Fitzgerald had had to do when Minnie was younger.

In 1877, pretty Lizzie Maddern died. Within the year, Minnie was touring in *A Messenger from Jarvis Section.* She was 13 and on her own, except for occasional visits to her Aunt Emma. Fortunately she was a likeable girl and an excellent actress, and there was no shortage of parts. Her only difficulty seemed to be in keeping her clothes on:

> Barney MacAuley was a nervous actor who believed that a star would be "wrapped in the solitude of his own originality." Minnie played a muted Clip and tried not to divert attention from the star, but her daydreaming and carelessness about her clothes were her undoing, and MacAuley's. Sometimes he would find the attention of the audience had deserted him for Minnie Maddern, who was absentmindedly stepping out of a petticoat or some other garment which had come off at the wrong moment.
>
> After such a mishap, MacAuley would have an agonizing scene with Minnie.
>
> "Miss Maddern, is it impossible for you to keep your clothes on?" and failing to get any convincing reassurance, he would end with the despairing admonition: "Lock your clothes on! Bolt them on!!"[2]

Her mind was on other things, not unnatural in a 14 year old.

When she was 16, Joe Havlin, who had helped her join MacAuley, proposed that she star in *Fogg's Ferry*, an amateur playwright's imitation of the kind of thing Lotta Crabtree was having such a success with. He wanted to take it straight to New York. Now, Minnie knew that she was not Lotta, but she also knew that a New York debut as a star was a fortunate opportunity, so she accepted the role. The critics, including 20 year old Harrison Grey Fiske of *The Dramatic Mirror* and the youngest editor in New York, were entranced with Miss Maddern, while universally condemning the play. Audiences loved Minnie *and* the play, and the 16 year old found herself a genuine star! She was very pretty and very popular, and in an amusing foreshadowing of events to come, Charles Frohman and David Belasco came to fisticuffs over the chance to be the first to present her with flowers. What more could a girl ask?

The answer, of course, was "romance," and Lagrande White, a musician, was only too ready to supply that. He toured with her and courted her through every city and hamlet on the circuit. When they returned to to New York, they were engaged. White's family was prominent in the piano business and he intended to star his bride in a new show with his family's backing. Minnie had quite definite ideas of what and who, especially who, she wanted in the show, and nothing would do for her, but the most expensive leading man in New York to support her. Eventually the play opened and was a minor success, although it closed rather quickly. So did the marriage. Soon the ex–Mrs. White was touring again.

She spent the weeks between tours with her Aunt Emma in Larchmont. There she renewed her acquaintance with Harrison Grey Fiske, the young editor who had been so smitten with her earlier efforts. The friendship ripened into courtship and then into an engagement. It became a legendary marriage. When the time came for her second nuptials, Minnie had been doing some hard thinking. She blamed the theatre and her involvement in it for breaking up her first marriage. This time, she decided to take no chances, and announced her retirement. After the honeymoon which was snowbound and tense, the young couple returned to New York and Minnie applied herself assiduously to learning housekeeping. She sent to Brentano's for a complete set of books on the subject (perhaps those by Mrs. Mowatt), and set to work. Alas, this was one play whose lines she couldn't seem to master, and Harrison had to take over the day-to-day management of their home. Minnie began to regret her departure from the world where she had been a success. Matters between the couple became even more strained when she expressed no desire for children. Perhaps that should be phrased differently. She expressed a desire for *no* children. Harrison Fiske was a conventionally reared young man for all his stagestruck ways, and he was taken aback. In his world, a young wife axiomatically became a young mother.

Once he realized that Minnie was adamant, he encouraged her to return to the theatre for a limited engagement in his play *Hester Crewe*. The play was a failure, financially (Fiske had acted as producer as well), and artistically. Nonetheless, when she was asked to do it again as a benefit, she balked at resurrecting *Hester* again. Instead, she suggested that the performance of *A Doll's House* by Henrik Ibsen. The play had first been brought to her attention by Laurence Barratt, but she hadn't cared for it. It didn't even seem to her to be a play. It was only three acts long and nothing much happened in it. When Barrett died, his obituary recorded his disappointment that he had failed to interest a single American actress in the play. Barrett was an old friend of the Maddern family and Minnie felt personally reproached by the comment. As she read the play again periodically during the early years of her marriage, she began to understand it better.

During her years on the stage, she had begun to formulate a theory about acting that was antithetical to the practices of the time. She began to abhor the heightened emotionalism then rampant in the theatre. Actors literally and figuratively chewed the scenery and actresses sometimes threw themselves on the stage floor and rolled about in an excess of passion. Minnie came to feel that all this was unnecessary.

> Although she had been trained in the old repertory or stock-company system, learning to play standard roles from the older actors, she saw that this training was largely useless for the new drama whose characters were not conceived in the traditional lines. She looked to life off the stage and to the new science of psychology for guidance in acting the new characters of realistic drama. She played with her back to the audience. She threw away lines. She substituted the eloquence of realistic posture and movement for the eloquence of language.[3]

The failure of *Hester Crewe*, which she'd played along standard lines, freed her somewhat. So did the nature of the event at which *A Doll's House* was presented. The benefit matinee was a one-shot performance with an audience drawn, not from the theatre, but from charitable society. One suspects that Minnie Maddern Fiske felt that with this audience she would be risking little and that no one of any theatrical consequence would know of her experimental production. She couldn't have been more wrong.

Ibsen wrote from Norway, commending her courage in undertaking his play. The audience, which had heard that Ibsen was dark and unapproachable, was charmed by her childlike, laughing, first-act "Nora," and followed her transformation with breathless anticipation. Within days, word of Mrs. Fiske's astounding performance had reached the highest theatrical circles and audiences were clamoring for her return to the theatre.

Harry Fiske recognized the inevitable. His Minnie was an actress, not a wife. He loved her dearly and he wanted the best for her so he supported her full-fledged return to the stage. She began a touring season of repertory, while Harry looked for *the play*. In time he sent her Thomas Hardy's dramatic adaptation of his novel *Tess of the D'Urbervilles*. She agreed that the script, or rather the book on which it was based, had real possibilities, but Hardy's script was unplayable. They located a playwright and began to work on the script. The production was fraught with perils. The Fiskes' partner and producer, Charles Lee, went bankrupt and they tempted fate with the leading actors they engaged, including an unreliable leading man, notorious for missing performances, and a dipsomaniac. Nevertheless, like many other actors across the years, the two, Charles Cochrane and Edward Bell, gave the performances of their careers when supporting Mrs. Fiske. In addition, Cochrane missed not one performance and Bell was sober for the entire run.

All of their friends warned them against doing the play, pointing to its "unnatural" heroine, who, they were sure, would be repulsive to the audience. Aunt Emma Maddern appealed to Minnie's "womanly modesty" not to portray the degenerate Tess, but her niece refused to be dissuaded.

Despite all the advice and the misfortune *Tess* opened. Perhaps there will never be another opening night to equal it. The audience rose in a body to applaud and the critics were euphoric. Most of the encomiums were reserved for Mrs. Fiske. Never, they declared, had such an actress been seen in the theatre! She was acclaimed the greatest actress of the nineteenth century:

> Mrs. Fiske's *Tess* is a personation of tremendous intensity and startling realism. Its emotional phases are expressed with the utmost quietness, but with a power that never fails to reach the heart of the most unimpressible spectator. It is a marvellous exhibition of the inherent force of suppression. The crescendo in Mrs. Fiske's characterization is remarkable; there is constantly increasing suspense and continually growing emotional force until the break comes just after the murder of Alec.[4]

The murder was an incredible emotional moment, and it revealed Mrs. Fiske's growing artistry. She challenged the "old ways" of the stage, particularly at the moment

> . . . when Tess murdered Alec D'Urberville. She walked out of the room. . . . The stage was empty. Then came the long wait while the audience — keyed up to high excitement — listened for an outcry. There was not a sound. At last Tess came back — and you saw in her face that she had killed Alec.
> This scene . . . had been thought impossible by practical people of the theatre . . . they warned the actress that no one could hold an audience so long with an empty stage. But she did. She made everybody believe in the thing that was going on beyond the door.[5]

Tess was Mrs. Fiske's first great role. She played it to sold-out houses in New York for months and then took it on the road. This first road tour brought to a head the worsening relations between the Theatrical Trust and the Fiskes.

In the early 1890s, before the creation of the Trust during the 1895–96 season, theatrical conditions in the hinterlands were somewhat chaotic. In every town there were one or two theatres, much as there are small movie houses across America today. Each season, the owner or manager of these houses came to New York to arrange the attractions which would appear in his theatre for the following year. Competition was open and the theatres paid as little, and the actors demanded as much, as they could. Eventually the "combination" grew up. A combination was an amalgamation of most of the first class theatres in a district which would band together to make a "circuit" of attractions. The owners would book attractions through a single agent in New York. Quickly, entrepreneurial businessmen saw the opportunities that could arise from controlling a "combination of the combinations," and that is just what theatre owners Sam Nixon and Fred Zimmerman of Philadelphia, and Al Hayman and Charles Frohman of New York, did when they joined wth booking agents Marc Klaw and Abe Erlanger of New York. They effectively owned both ends of the supply and demand continuum by booking acts and owning or controlling the theatres which presented the acts. By eliminating the demands of the marketplace, they could control the price. It was very tidy — if you were the one doing the the controlling and less so, if you were on the other end — which is where Mrs. Fiske found herself. It was also very profitable. Frohman alone, during the first decade of the 20th century, owned theatres in New York and London worth millions of dollars, and made a payroll of $35,000,000 a year to 10,000 employess — actors, stagehand, directors, etc. His advertising budget was an astounding $500,000 — then there were no electronic media to spend it on.[6]

Theoretically these combinations should have benefited actors by guaranteeing them a number of performances at a fixed salary. Unfortunately, the quality of the productions declined quickly when artistic considerations were waived aside in favor of the numerical balances in a ledger, and when actors' salary demands were not met because there was no competition for their performances.

> [T]he venerable William Winter exclaimed that the theatre had "passed from the hands of those who ought to control it — the hands of Actors who love and honor their art or of men endowed with the temperament of the Actor and acquainted with his art and its needs, — and, almost entirely, it has fallen into the clutches of sordid money-grubbing tradesmen, who have turned it into a bazaar."[7]

The Trust bought up or bribed any independent theatres which threatened to produce rival attractions. In short order, they controlled "the road," and most actors: "they turned the owners of out-of-town theatres into janitors of their buildings, subject, for the year's attractions, to the dictates of the Trust.[8]

At first Harrison Grey Fiske remained neutral on the issue, merely reporting in *the Dramatic Mirror* the purchases of theatres and such events as the forced reduction in salary demands of stars like Mme. Janauschak — and later her forced retirement. The Trust took exception to the *Mirror's* comments and forbade Harrison to mention them in his paper. They also attempted to bar any actors in their employ from reading the paper or advertising in it. Gradually matters worsened and Erlanger and Fiske actually came to blows on a New York street one afternoon.

There were actors who refused to accept the demands of the Trust. Their leader was Richard Mansfield, and their members included James O'Neill, Francis Wilson, James Hearne, and Minnie Maddern Fiske. Mansfield was bribed to join the Trust and the infant opposition group, the Independent Theatre Artists, fell apart.[9] By the end of 1898 only Francis Wilson stood with Minnie and in January of 1899, he too, had succumbed. Eventually only Mrs. Fiske was left to stand against the Syndicate. She toured *Tess*, going into any city where she could find a theatre to take her, playing in third-rate theatres that hadn't had a legitimate drama in a generation. The clamor to see Mrs. Fiske in her notorious play was so great that she played to S.R.O. houses wherever she appeared.

> Mrs. Fiske . . . was justly adored by a tremendous national public as the incarnation of honesty and valor. The theatre, is inevitably art by committee and compromise, but Mrs. Fiske struck bargains with no one on earth. Besides being possibly the greatest and most versatile actress of her day, she was a tireless foe of the Theatre Trust known as the Syndicate and an articulate champion of causes. (She once had a man arrested for mistreating a horse.)[10]

The following season she and Harrison brought together a young playwright and *Vanity Fair*. From Thackeray's lively novel they fashioned *Becky Sharp* as a starring vehicle for Mrs. Fiske. The play opened in Montreal and ran most of the night. Reviews were disastrous and the Syndicate gleefully ran reprints of them in the New York papers and assumed that that finished the opposition. The Fiskes, however, had no other play to present that season, so they worked frantically to get *Becky* into shape and then limped into New York with it. The opening was brilliant and the cast took 12 curtain calls. Mrs. Fiske's hold on the American stage was even more firmly established. The show ran in Manhattan until the manager was forced to close it to bring in another play to which he had a commitment, and Minnie took *Becky* on tour.

The Syndicate's stranglehold on theatres was tightening but Harry worked diligently to find obscure or long closed houses whose bewildered owners suddenly found themselves hosts to the first lady of the American theatre. On this tour, Minnie was determined to go west, beyond Chicago, and to do it she played in vaudeville houses and in tents. But wherever she went, audiences followed while the Syndicate gnashed its teeth. By this time she was fighting them virtually alone.

In Denver in 1899, while on tour with *Becky Sharp*, Mrs. Fiske was reduced to playing a dime-a-seat house in the slums with a tiny stage, "the size of a parlor."[11] One of the most famous scenes in the play took place during the Second Act in a large ballroom. Throughout the First Act, the audience had buzzed with speculation. How could Mrs. Fiske stage this legendary setting? When the curtain rose, the ballroom was there, in its entirety. It wasn't until a brisk December draft prompted the audience to huddle into their coats that they realized that the back wall of the theatre had been removed to accommodate the scenery. Mrs. Fiske's audience *always* got their money's worth!

Sometimes the Trust diverted rival attractions to perform against her, and she had the dubious pleasure of appearing against erstwhile allies, like James O'Neill in *The Count of Monte Cristo*. Generally she outdrew them.

From New York, though, Harry sent good news. He had obtained the lease of a theatre in Manhattan through a loophole and closed the deal before the Trust discovered the true identity of the new management. When Mrs. Fiske came off the road this time, she'd have a new theatre to go into.

Once again in New York, Minnie abandoned her usually strong theatrical instincts and appeared in two finds of Harry's. They were two society "dramas" and were as outmoded as the Victorian morality they espoused. Wisely Mrs. Fiske revived *Tess* and played once more to sold-out houses for weeks.

The following season, the Fiskes presented *Mary of Magdala*, ghost-translated by William Winter, with a cast of 150 and costarring Tyrone Power as Judas. Audiences filed out after the curtain as if they had been in church and ministers praised the production from the pulpit. It ran for an entire season. Minnie took it to theatres open to her in the East and was contemplating a European tour when Tyrone Power announced his departure for other roles. Although Mrs. Fiske had always been largely responsible for the staging of her plays, with *Mary of Magdala* she assumed the true role of director: "As a stage director . . . she tried to develop expert ensemble playing in which small parts were as well acted as the large parts, and in which each actor served the overall design of the play. She believed in giving special attention to the weaker sections of the play so that the whole drama would be strengthened."[12]

Particularly notable about the production of *Mary of Magdala* was Mrs. Fiske's handling of the crowd scenes. Each super was individually selected, coached, given a character and actions. Critics particularly praised the flavor of the crowd scenes, finding them reminiscent of true life in the east.

> In directing her actors, Mrs. Fiske worked tirelessly to develop their awareness of psychological truth. She demanded that her players have a reason for every movement they made and for every speech they uttered. In rehearsals she carefully explained the circumstances of each scene, the state of mind of each character and then the company worked out the business which seemed logical and appropriate for the scene. Once the action and the details were decided on, they were rehearsed until they fitted perfectly into the smooth flow of the drama. Mrs. Fiske's advice to her company was: "Take plenty of time. Don't hurry. Tremendous situations, wonderful emotions, great events do not rush. They are like the mills of the gods, grinding slowly but exceedingly small," . . . Beatrice Sturges . . . after watching her direct a rehearsal, wrote: "Nothing is too small for the eye and the attention of Mrs. Fiske — whether it be the gesture of an actor, a detail in stage setting or lighting, a tone of voice, or a strain of music — and it is her watchful care and artistic sense that have made her company a model one to see."[13]

Veteran performer that she was, Minnie "had a horror of boring the audience. So at rehearsals she believed in working hardest on the dullest protions of a play; they must be made to hold attention."[14]

Minnie Maddern Fiske also served as what is now called an artistic director overseeing all aspects of the production. "[S]he ran her shows from top to bottom, poking her actors as one goads a slow-burning fire, charging around back stage to check on morale . . . drilling the ushers."[15]

Her success convinced her that New York and her company were ready for the ultimate test. In the fall the Manhattan Theatre presented *Hedda Gabler*. Critics were outraged by the play, but once again they were entranced by Mrs. Fiske's portrayal.

> Mrs. Fiske was intellectual and analytical by nature. . . . Before acting a character, she believed in understanding both his mind and his heart and in knowing the reason or impulse which prompted his words or actions. . . . She included only those elements which fulfilled the overall design . . . each detail counted; every gesture and tone had significance. . . . The actress suggested rather than exhibited the emotions of her characters and thus gained powerful effects. . . .[16]

Her Hedda was icy and catlike and cruel. It was not a "pretty" play or a "pretty" performance, but it was devastatingly modern:

> [S]he had taught audiences to listen to Ibsen and like it. To her, these plays were tales about very real, comprehensible people; besides she could see witty implications in the lines. So her Ibsen performances had a crisp astringent humor interwoven with the tragic themes — a happy surprise to people who had come braced for gloom."[17]

With her production of *Hedda Gabler* we may mark the true birth of 20th-century theatre. "Mrs. Fiske's artistic ideals and style of acting were necessary corollaries of the kinds of plays she preferred to produce."[18] Once again Minnie went on tour with *Hedda* while Harry produced a rapid succession of failures at the Manhattan. In 1904, a scheme they had thought about for several years was decided upon. The Manhattan Theatre would house a *permanent* theatre company. How Mrs. John Drew would have laughed at this *new* idea. Nevertheless, Minnie went forward with it while Harry recuperated from a life-threatening bout with typhoid fever.

They opened the season with *Becky Sharp* which was well received again. Mrs. Fiske was determined that all members of the company be shown to advantage. George Arliss was a young actor with the company and he told this story years later in his autobiography *Up the Years from Bloomsbury*:

> Our greatest difficulty was to prevent her from effacing herself. She was so interested in getting the best out of everybody else that she always seemed to regard herself as a negligible quantity in the play.
> I remember saying to her, "Are you going to speak all that with your back to the audience?"
> "Yes," she said, "I want them to see your face."
> "But," I remonstrated, "it's a very long speech for you to deliver in that position."
> "Yes, I know," she sighed. "It's such a long speech that I want to get through with it as quickly as I can."[19]

In December, they premiered *Leah Kleschna*, a play ideally cast from their company. By now Minnie was directing and producing as well as acting. The critics at first were enthralled, declaring the play "too great to have been written by an American." In later reviews, reason returned and with it the recognition that *Leah Kleschna* was essentially a melodrama. It didn't matter to the audiences. The play ran till June to packed houses. The expected tour did not materialize that summer. The Trust had bought up, and, in many cases, closed the strings of second and third rate theatres where Minnie had been appearing. The East was now also closed to her.

In September, matters had changed. While the Syndicate was concentrating on closing out the single actress who opposed them, the Shubert brothers and David Belasco had each been buying individual theatres as they became available. Almost overnight two dozen first-class houses were available for a Fiske tour. There was only one difficulty. The fledgling Shubert empire was precarious and heavily mortgaged and they were counting on the drawing power of Mrs. Fiske on tour to enable them to hang onto their newly acquired network. She could do nothing but agree to help them in their mutual fight against the tyrannical Trust. Accordingly, the Manhattan Theatre Company was reformed to tour rather than open a New York season. *Leah Kleschna* was revived for this purpose and the company housed in a special railroad car. For the first time in years, Minnie Maddern Fiske was touring to first-rate theatres and in a manner which befitted her stature in the theatre. "No other actress had made such a tour, breaking records in cities and barnstorming at crossroads; fighting for survival with one hand, and the freedom of the theatre with the other."[20]

Minnie was a tiny woman with her father's red hair and her mother's enormous eyes. "The eyes of Minnie Maddern Fiske are the chief allurements in her face. They are big and oval, with sensitive lids, and long lashes. They change color and vibrate with every mood."[21]

Because the theatre was an emotional world, she had a surfeit of it and avoided it in her private life.

> Mrs. Fiske never made a display of emotion off the stage, keeping her steady, glinting humor on the surfacce. She was not a disorganized genius, but a well-balanced one. Her attitude was impersonal, even toward herself. The only thing that betrayed her was her intense pity for neglected wretched animals. In every town on tour she knew the way to the dog-and-cat hospital, and many a starving kitten had its board bill paid by her.[22]

She was a woman who tried to give up the theatre, only to realize that it was only in that world that she felt comfortable. Once she came to that awareness, she threw herself totally into her work. "The power and clarity of her acting came from the power and clarity of her mind. Hers was always a gallant spirit. As she grew older, she never indulged in self-pity or a backward glance."[23] Regrets were for those who were afraid of the future, and Minnie thought she feared nothing the years to come would bring.

In 1905, the Fiskes decided to relinquish the Manhattan Theatre, but to retain the Manhattan Theatre company. The play they chose for that season was *The New York Idea* by Langdon Mitchell, a comical satire on divorce. Like Mrs. Fiske's other hits, it played well to adoring audiences, and she took it on tour. Despite the inroads the Shuberts had made on the Trust's organization, all the theatres west of Chicago that truly deserved the name were closed to the Fiske tour, but she pressed on playing places like Yanton, South Dakota, and Raton, New Mexico Territory, where there was a rollerskating rink, but no theatre and no houses. It didn't matter. A makeshift stage was erected in the rink and chairs and benches were borrowed from all over. The audience came by horseback and buggy from miles around. Most had never seen live entertainment before and a sophisticated comedy about divorce was very removed from their own experiences. Nonetheless, they were an enthusiastic and appreciative audience.

En route, the company rail car was unhitched from the train and left standing miles from civilization (the blackguards of the Syndicate were suspected). No matter — another locomotive arrived hours later and accommodatingly raced them across the desert to make their El Paso curtain.

On this tour, she played more than one skating rink. There were also deserted theatres occupied by bats, churches, town halls, and outdoor arenas where the actors had to dress in nearby homes. *This* was the tour which evolved out of a "cracked" Trust. For Minnie it was enough that she could appear in towns that had been "Trust territory" for more than a decade.

Harry Fiske, in New York, believed that his wife's popularity would continue to soar and that she would attract audiences forever. Minnie knew better. From Waterloo, Iowa, she wrote him:

> [W]e must see the danger if we do not begin to accumulate *now*. We must put by money as soon as we are able . . . I am now nearly forty-two years of age. The little popularity I have may wane . . . I have a horror of an old age of financial distress and all the humiliation it brings. Let us determine to avoid it. . . . There is danger in delay of this resolve—I do not speak in the slightest spirit of gloom or depression. Not in the least. It is only that we must devote ourselves to protecting the future.[24]

She needn't have bothered to write. Harry was too busy sending out failing companies to pay much attention.

The years, the tours, the productions rolled on . . . Ibsen's *Rosmersholm*, Edward Sheldon's *Salvation Nell*, Gerhard Hauptmann's *Hannele*, and Ibsen's *Pillars of Society* . . .

Salvation Nell was a gritty portrayal of life in the slums with Mrs. Fiske almost unrecognizable as Nell, a scrubwoman.[25]

In defending Nell as his property, Jim Platt kills a man, and before the police arrive, Nell sits on the floor holding her drunken lover's head in her lap for fully ten minutes without a word, almost without a motion. The barroom was the scene of hurried activity but, gradually one could watch nothing else; one became absorbed in the silent pathos of that dumb sitting figure. Miss Mary Garden, herself a distinguished actress, said of this, "Ah, to be able to *do nothing* like that!"[26]

Once, when speaking of her method, Mrs. Fiske said "For months before I attempt even to rehearse a part and many weeks before I begin to study the words assigned for me to say, I am imagining myself to be the character to be assumed."[27]

As she had been doing for so many years, Mrs. Fiske took *Nell* on tour during the summer. This tour marked the climax of Minnie's fight with the Syndicate. While appearing at the Lyric Theatre in Cincinnati, Minnie Maddern Fiske received a telegram which waved the white flag.

The telegram was from the New York City office of Charles Frohman, and it offered Mrs. Fiske the use of any Syndicate house which she cared to occupy, on independent term; all the theatres of America were open to her, and her days of barnstorming in churches and skating rinks were over.

The Trust that had surrendered to a woman had recently controlled all the theatres in America; it had a firm hold in England and Australia, and it reached tentacles into France and Germany. For years Mrs. Fiske had stood alone against the Trust, a pinpoint of resistance. But the pinpoint was diamond hard, and with the weight of the Shuberts and Belasco behind it, it had split the Trust.[28]

In later years, she would even appear under the management of Klaw and Erlanger, and she lived long enough to see her erstwhile allies, the Shuberts, become as monopolistic as her old enemies.

The great 12-year ordeal, playing in honky-tonk houses and ghost-theatres, had taken its toll. If it had broken the trust it had also broken Mrs. Fiske; she was exhausted, worn out, and nearly penniless.

In New York, Harry continued to produce, sometimes great successes like *Kismet* starring Otis Skinner, more often great failures like *The White Dove* starring a retired ballerina. Harry was in love with the idea of the theatre. Mrs. Fiske's major biographer, Archie Binns, suggests in his book that the Fiskes were a kind of latter-day Macbeths. She, drawn to the theatre, entices her husband into new and foreign paths until he is consumed by theatrical passions and she, regretful, wishes to retreat.[29] It seems a labored and extended metaphor for what were probably the inevitable consequences of a marriage between a great actress and a stagestruck journalist.

The years of battle with the Trust were over but Minnie's combative spirit never rested. With each passing year she became more involved with the work of the Humane Society. For years, wherever she toured, she was notorious for surrounding herself with abused, mistreated, and abandoned animals which she picked up, nursed back to health, and foisted off on friends whenever possible. Her campaigns were extended to help carriage and cartage horses, and cattle on their way to market. She fought successfully for closed cattle cars and to provide the beasts with food and water on their journey to the slaughterhouse. Mrs. Fiske passionately opposed bull fighting and clubbing seals for their fur, but her greatest triumph came as the saviour of the snowy egret. Normally, she was extremely wary of publicity and personal promotion, but she threw her entire being into the cause of preventing the extinction of the birds. Their very fashionable feathers could only be obtained by killing the female as she cared for her young. Experts had already written off the egret, consigning it to the same fate as the passenger pigeon, when Mrs. Fiske began her impassioned defense. Society women were shamed into joining her cause, and within a single season, the fashion for egret feathers had become démodé. Laws were passed to ensure that the birds would always be protected. Other environmental concerns, begun by Theodore Roosevelt, were also given enormous impetus by this victory. The birds made a near-miraculous recovery from certain extinction, and within a few years were removed from endangered lists.

Over the next decade, the star which had shone so favorably over Mrs. Fiske flickered occasionally. For every prodigious hit like *Mrs. Bumpstead-Leigh*, there were several failures, sometimes several in the same season. With the superstition engrained in all troupers, Minnie expected a failure for every success and her long run of hits had awakened a fear of a longer run of failures.

She repeatedly urged Harry to conserve their resources and squirrel away funds against her dread of a penniless old age, but he didn't share her presentiments of the long, dry years to come. The late twenties were a difficult time for the Fiskes in many ways. Harry followed up a successful production of *The Merry Wives of Windsor* with Otis Skinner and Mrs. Fiske with a lavish production of *Much Ado About Nothing* on which he squandered all his skill and care and money. Again Mrs. Fiske was the star. It was not until *Much Ado* had played for some weeks that Harry analyzed its revenue and production expenses and discovered that even sold-out houses would lose money. It was a devastating revelation. Eventually the Fiskes lost $100,000 on the production. It was a loss they were never able to recoup. Mrs. Fiske found her nightmare of a penniless old age, playing diminshed roles in third rate companies, no longer an improbability.

To add to her woes, Emily Stevens, her younger first cousin, died in 1928 of a combination of pneumonia brought on by exposure, and an overdose of sleeping pills. Emily was the daughter Mrs. Fiske had never had, and a skilled and versatile actress in her own right. That same year, Mary

Maddern, the last of "The Singing Maddern Sisters," died and with her went the final remnants of Minnie Maddern Fiske's fragmented but cherished childhood. For the first time, Minnie felt her own advancing years weigh on her.

Her natural conservatism kept the Fiskes out of the stock market, so the crash in '29 only affected her indirectly. Her then current vehicle, *Ladies of the Jury*, opened on October 21, 1929, with one of those legendary traffic jams of moneyed theatregoers who only a week later would be caught in their own tragedies. The night was golden, the play enthusiastically received, the star hailed. And it all ended a few days later when the management closed the play for fear that the audiences would be affected by the growing depression.

In March of the following year, she played a limited run as Mrs. Malaprop in a revival of her famous production of *The Rivals*. No one knew it then, but it would be her last appearance on a New York stage.

Mrs. Fiske continued to perform for the remainder of her life. She longed to retire from the stage and put away forever her make-up and costumes, but she was simply unable to do so. There was no money.

In 1930, despite Harry's protests, she accepted a flat $600 a week for six weeks in California. Times were hard, and she knew the offer was as good as could be hoped for.

George Taylor, her old manager, put together a small company and sent them on the road. His idea was a novel one. The audiences of each city would vote on which of Mrs. Fiske's great hits they wanted to see and the company would perform accordingly. The troupe limped across the country and then home, and Mrs. Fiske returned poorer than ever. Almost all of her proceeds had been pumped back into the tour to keep the company afloat.

When she returned, she went at last to see a physician. The frightening, unexplained pains which had dogged her across the country were solved and the explanation was more frightening than the pains. Harry kept the diagnosis of cancer from her, but she wrote her will and prepared for her last play. *Against the Wind* by Carlos Drake might instead have been titled *Against All Odds*. Two weeks before it was to open she collapsed and her doctor absolutely forbade her to continue. Her dear friend Henrietta Crosman agreed to take the role, sight unseen, as a favor to Minnie, and the play went to Rochester and Cleveland, where it faltered badly. Minnie read the reviews, gathered her strength and set off for Cleveland where she rejoined the cast. It seemed impossible to the actors that she would be able to perform. She had to rest constantly in an armchair in the wings between scenes, and she was unquestionably frail.

In Chicago she nearly collapsed on stage and the critics could not, would not, review the performance, as they thought of a woman dying on stage. Miraculously, Minnie began to rally and as she improved, so did the play. By the end of the run, she seemed so much better, she was able to send Harry and Carlos Drake on to New York with light words.

> Holding out both her hands, she told them gaily. "You wouldn't believe me, would you two? Well, most people have to be shown before they'll believe anything!"
>
> It was not renewed strength Minnie had discovered — only the way of giving her ultimate reserves. When they were gone, she drove herself by force of will alone, to the end of her sixteenth Chicago performance. In hypnotized awe, her last audiences watched two plays by the same name acted on one stage. The slight comedy with many characters, and the more somber play with only one, a small determined dying woman, beating against the wind of eternity.[30]

From Chicago, she returned to New York completely done in. She was put to bed at the home of her secretary, Mae Cox, and a doctor summoned. He examined her closely and declared that she had been misdiagnosed. She suffered not from cancer, but from intestinal poisoning and exhaustion. The exhaustion had strained her heart and that was now the critical problem. She spent the next two months sleeping and seemed to improve, but on February 14, 1932, her heart gave out. "Like the creatures she had so often befriended, she crawled off to die quickly, without any fuss made over it."[31] There would be no more performances.

After her death, the critics debated her place in the history of the stage. Was she, with Duse, Bernhardt, and Terry, the last great actress of the legitimate theatre, or was she, as George Jean Nathan proclaimed, "not an actress at all?"

> Robert Garland . . . referred to her as "The Great Lady of the Theatre, the High Class Low Comedienne, the Grand Old Trouper," who, in his "Prejudiced and unreliable eyes," could do no wrong. "She could star herself in a dramatization of the telephone directory and I would praise her. For there is something about her which delights me, something I have never been able to get into words." She is an excellent example of that sort of actress who confuses and confounds the standards of criticism, rendering indistinguishable from each other the technique of acting and the display of personal mannerisms.[32]

John Rankin Towse had no such difficulties. To his mind, Minnie Maddern Fiske was *not* an actress.

> The very essence of acting to my mind, lies in the capacity of assumption and impersonation of a conceived character and personality different from that of the player. Perfect metamorphosis, in body and spirit, is an idealism very rarely, if ever, possible of achievement, . . . in all her "creations" [Mrs. Fiske] had presented her own identity without any substantial modification of speech, gesture, look or manner. Situations, circumstances differed, but not the personality. It may be granted unreservedly that the personality was uncommon, piquant, provocative, and interesting and exceedingly effective in parts with which it happened to be in accordance. . . . Her elocution was faulty and did not lend itself

readily to emotional expression. She could be imperious, sarcastic, fiery, and angry, but the deeper notes of passion she could not sound, and her pathos was hard and hollow, without the true ring.[33]

But she had her defenders. Like Robert Garland, William Winter, the critic, was one.

> She has a personality so distinct, so exquisitely spiritistic and original that all the graces of her art are subservient to her own individuality. Her face is a delightful cameo mask out of which shine deep intellecutality and sympathy, keenly artistic temperament, and a genius that is elemental in its delicate force.[34]

Winter and Towse differ fundamentally in their definition of acting and in that difference lies the real unresolvable debate about Mrs. Fiske as an actress. Although they and their fellows did not realize it, when they argued the merits of Minnie's performances and personality, they were really discussing the coming of age of the theatre. Despite the fact that nearly all of her most successful plays were produced before World War I, Minnie Maddern Fiske was the ultimate 20th century actress. There was little of the "old school" when she appeared on the stage. Thoroughly familiar with the traditional techniques of the 19th century, she chose to reject them in favor of new, untried and uncertain techniques which felt right, but which were completely foreign to most of her fellow performers. With Mrs. Fiske, the theatre matured, and was able to look forward to experimentation and naturalism with complete confidence in "the Modern School." It was Mrs. Fiske's gift to the future.

In his book *Three Hundred Years of American Acting*, Garff Wilson provides a masterly summary of Minnie Maddern Fiske's career and its effects on the theatre.

> Of all the influences which helped rejuvenate the American theatre, none is more important than Minnie Maddern Fiske. Her role as a pioneer is often overlooked. Although she is rarely given credit for being an innovator, her career marks a clean break with the traditions of the nineteenth century and the emergence of those ideals which dominate the stage of our time. She was a champion of the works of Ibsen. . . . She depreciated the star system and tried to develop a company of players in which the individual was subordinate to the ensemble. . . . Most significant of all, she advocated a simple natural style of acting based on psychological truthfulness and freedom from theatrical trickery. . . . Mrs. Fiske exerted strong influence on the stage as an actress, a manager and a stage director. As a manager she fought the Theatrical Syndicate. . . . As a stage manager she adopted many of the practices of the modern regisseur. . . . She illustrated in both her acting and her directing many ideals and techniques which are still dominant; and . . . she was a pioneer who contributed significantly to the theatrical renaissance of the twentieth century[35]

For 45 years, Minnie Maddern Fiske had been in the forefront of her profession, the acknowledged "First Lady of the American Theatre." For more than a decade she'd fought for the conscience of the theatre, dreading the decline which seemed inevitable under the mass-produced fodder of the Syndicate. Ultimately she won that war and the defeat of the Trust changed American theatre forever. However, Mrs. Fiske's most enduring contribution was one she would have been proud to acknowledge. Minnie Maddern Fiske made a profound alteration in the very fabric of the theatre itself. She invented the "art of not acting" years before Stanislavski gave character study a good name:

> [B]efore the theories of the Moscow Art Theatre gained currency in America, Minnie Maddern Fiske was teaching similar principles and applying them in her productions. . . . Her ideals and methods reached maturity as early as 1897, and she organized her Manhattan Theatre Company in 1904 to demonstrate her theories of acting and play production. The Moscow Art Theatre was not founded until 1898, and the first Russian-trained player to perform in the United States did not appear until 1905.[36]

She rescued Ibsen from early obscurity and in the process changed the kind of plays done on the American stage. Essentially Minnie Maddern Fiske developed a school of acting which can be thought of as psychologically modern in scope and intent. She emphasized the actor's search for the underlying psychological truths of his character and sought to eliminate any movement not motivated by internal feelings. In contrast to the highly stylized and very popular 19th-century "stage speech," she demanded vocal and physical "reality" from her performers in their characterizations. Finally, Mrs. Fiske was concerned with presenting the playwright's vision on the stage. Not for her the rearrangement of a play to create "points," or to showcase a particular actor or talent. If an actor was unsuitable for a role, he was not cast. The actor was to adapt to the play rather than adapting the play to the actor. It was a revelation to theatregoers to see a carefully presented, wholly realized, and integrated performance.[37]

Her company emphasized "the ensemble" decades before "the group" or "method acting" became popular, and, for her, the importance of giving each actor in a scene his "moment" while maintaining the unity of the production, outweighed any importance due to her for her stardom. Throughout her career, Mrs. Fiske remained far in the vanguard of current theatrical thinking. Her ideas were far more advanced than those of her compatriots, and it was only when common practice caught up with her innovations that the styles and methods which she had introduced became the standard currency of the stage.[38]

Mrs. Fiske was an actress of the 19th century who helped to create the theatre of the 20th. Every production today on Broadway, every play performed in repertory theatres across the country, and every amateur theatrical, every community theatre, contains a little of her legacy to the stage.

EPILOGUE

The leading ladies of the American stage have had determination and resolution to a disproportionate degree. Resourcefulness was practically a constituent requirement for success in the theatres and playhouses which dotted the country from Boston to New Orleans; from Charleston to St. Louis to California. Actors made do, or did without, creating illusions out of paint and cheesecloth and candles which they shared with an audience, often as eager to be fooled as they were to fool them. It was a grand conspiracy of dreams fed by a consuming hunger for diversion from the harsher realities of daily life.

In this atmosphere, almost anything could become possible, and if some leading ladies wanted to manage the theatres or champion causes, or write new plays, or challenge the wilderness of the West, or the equally daunting rigors of the Old World, well, in a world of possibilities, why not?

Sometimes it is important to look at the first people to attempt some unusual feat to determine what created that impetus to abandon the familiar and dare the undone. What accident of fate pushed them into the loneliness of singularity? Often the answer can only be that a combination of circumstances, personality, and fortune are the key. None of the women I've profiled *chose* to be the first to act in Pittsburgh, or the first to manage a theatre in Philadelphia, or the only one to defeat the syndicate in South Dakota.

Instead they found themselves at a unique juncture where personal experience married the moment and fate intervened — sometimes for good, often for ill. We may therefore examine the lives of those who challenged "the way it was done" to carve new careers for themselves and to advance the theatre as it took root in American soil, in order to learn from their examples.

Perhaps it is possible to say that the individual is unimportant and that the innovation or reform or effect would have emerged when the time was right, regardless of one person more or less.

If Laura Keene and Louisa Lane Drew had not lived, would there have been women managing theatres in the 19th century? If Anna Cora Mowatt and Susanna Rowson had never existed, would their shoes have been filled by other women playwrights? If Minnie Maddern Fiske had given in, would theatre today still be controlled by a handful of businessmen? If Fanny Kemble had chosen to ignore the plight of the Southern slaves, would we need a passport today to go to Georgia? If Sophia Turner and Charlotte Cushman had selected other outlets for their talents, would theatre be so very different today?

One school of thought would deny the questions without hesitation. Theirs is a dehumanizing dictum which ignores the role of the individual in the larger historical perspective. Actually, of course, the answer to these questions is no more knowable than to speculate on the future of electricity and the portable radio, had Edison and Marconi died as babes in arms.

What is possible is to examine the effect of a living person on an ageless entity. The theatre is as eternal as the life force. It has existed in some form since apes climbed down out of trees to gather around a fire and watch the shadows dance, and it will continue in some form long after our descendants' descendants have settled planets in the Andromeda galaxy. Wherever people gather together, there will be those who entertain — for fame, for fortune, for glory — and because it is in the nature of man to entertain and to be entertained. This is the heritage which carries the theatre forward.

The theatre of the future will be shaped by the theatre of today, and the theatre of today has been shaped by the theatre of the past. Theatre in our own time owes something to the valiant respectability of Mrs. Mowatt; to the wit and facile pen of Mrs. Rowson: to the single-minded craft of Charlotte Cushman; to the tragic management of Laura Keene; to the courageous determination of Mrs. Fiske; to the centuries of theatrical tradition engrained in Mrs. John Drew; to the valor and tenacity of Sophia Turner; and to the shocked sensibilities of Fanny Kemble.

Their lives added to the rich theatrical traditions of the American stage. Each of them was uniquely American in outlook and each altered the texture of stage history irrevocably. All too often, their contributions were slightly regarded during their lifetimes, and it is only with the vision of historical perspective that we can ascertain their true importance, yet without their efforts, the American theatre of the past would have been a poorer and less exciting place, and the modern theatre and the theatre of the future would be immeasurbly impoverished.

Appendix

"MRS. FISKE PREPARES THE ACTOR"

It is by scientific rather than purely artistic methods that triumphs are achieved or perfection is accomplished.

Anyone may achieve on some rare occasion an outburst of genuine feeling, a gesture of imperishable beauty, a ringing accent of truth; but your scientific actor knows how he did it. He can repeat it again and again and again. He can be depended on. Once he has thought out his role and found the means to express his thought, he can always remember the means.

...consider your voice; first, last and always your voice. It is the beginning and end of acting. Train that till it responds to your thought and purpose with absolute precision ... [Other necessities are] everything that makes for health, everything that makes for the fine *person*. Fresh air, for instance — fresh air, though you madden to murderous fury all the stuffy people ... with you.

And next your imagination. Use it.... An actor is exactly as big as his imagination ... and be reflective. Think.... Stay away from the theatre as much as you can.... Once become 'theatricalized' and you are lost.... Imagine a poet occupying his mind with the manners and customs of other poets, their plans, their methods, their prospects.... Dwell in this artificial world and you will know only the externals of acting.

Go into the streets, into the slums, into the fashionable quarters.... Become acquainted with sorrow, with many kinds of sorrow.... Go where you can find something fresh to bring back to the stage.... It is in the irony of things that the theatre should be the most dangerous place for the actor. But then, the world is the worst possible place, the most corrupting place for the human soul ... all of us can strive to remain uncontaminated. In the world, we must be unworldly; in the theatre the actor must be untheatrical....

Stay by yourself.... When a part comes to you, establish your own ideal for it, and, striving for that ... let nothing ... come between you and it. The test of acting is always "Is it true? Do people do this? The tone of mind must be true. Pay no attention to the other actors, unless they be real actors.... Unless it is a bitter matter of bread and butter, pay no attention or as little attention as possible to the director, unless he is a real director.... Above all, you must ignore the audience's very existence.

...no actor can afford to let the audience command him. He must be able to give as true a performance before three frigid persons as before a house packed to the brim with good will. That is his business.

If you have had a great night, if they have laughed and applauded and called you again and again before the curtain, accept their warming kindness gratefully, but on the way home ... ask yourself, "Did I really play well tonight?" ...turn to the critic within you and ask 'What was so very wrong with my performance tonight?'

— Adapted from *Mrs. Fiske, Her Views on the Stage*
by Alexander Woollcott

NOTES

Susanna Haswell Rowson

(Note: Sources are not given for statements which are generally accepted. Anyone interested in further material about Susanna Rowson is referred to the following books [for complete citations, see the Bibliography]: Nason, E., *A Memoir of Mrs. Susanna Rowson*; Parker, P.L., *Susanna Rowson*; Weil, D., *In Defense of Women, Susanna Rowson 1762–1824*; and Vail, R.W.G. *Susanna Rowson.*)

1. Elias Nason, *A Memoir of Mrs. Susanna Rowson* (Albany: Joel Munsell, 1870), pp. 5–9.

2. William S. Kable refutes this story in his preface to *Three American Novels* [including] *Charlotte: A Tale of Truth by Susannah Haswell Rowson*, Intro. by Wm. S. Kable (Columbus, Ohio: Charles E. Merrill, 1970). His assertion is that Otis was mad before he met young Susanna, and could not, therefore, have tutored her.

3. Nason, pp. 22–3.

4. With reference to her employer, Nason says merely, "A noble family," followed later by "her patron was Georgina, Duchess of Devonshire." Vail and Weil specifically state that Georgina was her employer, while Parker does not. Nason was the source closest to her own time period, and had access to her family and her papers, so it seems unlikely to me that he would have missed a noble connection.

5. Nason p. 34.

6. *Ibid.*, p. 34n.

7. Dorothy Weil, *In Defense of Women, Susanna Rowson 1762–1824*, (University Park and London: The Pennsylvania State University Press, 1976), p. 5.

8. *Ibid.*, p. 2.

9. Nason, pp. 118–19.

10. George O. Seilhamer, *A History of the American Theatre* (New York: Haskell House, 1969 reissue), Vol. 3, p. 143.

11. Julian Mates, *The American Musical Stage Before 1800* (New Brunswick: Rutgers Univ. Press, 1962), p. 189.

12. William Charvat, *The Profession of Authorship in America 1800–1870* (Columbus: Ohio State Univ. Press, 1968), p. 21.

13. Seilhamer, V.3, p. 150.

14. Mates, p. 161.

15. Mates, p. 189.

16. "A Defender of the Company" writing under the pen name of "Candid" in the Sept. 19, 1795, issue of the *Maryland Journal*, quoted in Robert W.G. Vail, *Susanna Haswell Rowson, the Author of Charlotte Temple, a Bibliographical Study*, American Antiquarian Society, New Series Vol. 42, 4/2/1932–10/19/1932 (Worcester: 1933), p. 53.

17. Seilhamer, V.3, p. 353.

18. *Ibid.*, V.3, p. 165.

19. Mates, p. 190.

20. Seilhamer, V.3, p. 155.

21. Vail, p. 144.

22. Arthur Hobson Quinn, *A History of the American Drama* (New York: F.S. Crofts, 1943), Vol. I, p. 181.

23. Seilhamer, V.3, p. 171.

24. *Ibid.*, Vol. 3, p. 352.

25. Apparently there was another actress by the name of Mrs. Rowson appearing at the turn of the 19th cetnury. The following story is taken from the 4/16/1801 issue of the *Norfolk Herald*, and quoted in Brooks McNamara, *The American Playhouse in the 18th Century* (Cambridge: Harvard Univ. Press, 1969): "It is recommended to the management to have regular examinations of the machinery below stage; for on Tuesday evening, owing to the ponderosity of Mrs. Rowson, the springs of a trap door gave way, and not only the leading lady disappeared, but she carried little Mrs. Stuart down also. A sailor in the pit observed, that it put him in mind of the 'Royal George' which when she went down, sucked a sloop of war into the vortex with her, that was at anchor at a little distance."

26. Mates, p. 189.

27. Weil, p. 4.

28. Joseph T. Buckingham, *Personal Memoirs and Recollections of Editorial Life* (Boston: n.p., 1852), Vol. 1, p. 85.

29. Clara M. Kirk and Rudolph Kirk, "Introduction," *Charlotte Temple, a Tale of Truth* (New York: Twayne, 1964), p. 14.

30. Charvat, p. 23.

31. Buckingham, V.1, p. 85.

32. Mates, p. 202.

33. Nason, pp. 102–3.

34. Vail, p. 59.

35. Buckingham, V.1, p. 85.

36. Nason, p. 193.

37. Charvat, p. 20.

38. *Ibid.*, p. 251.

Anna Cora Mowatt

(Note: Sources are not given for statements which are generally accepted. Anyone interested in further material about Anna Cora Mowatt Ritchie is referred to the following books [for complete citations, see the Bibliography]: Barnes, E., *The Lady of Fashion;* Mowatt, A.C., *Autobiography of an Actress;* and, although it is not strictly nonfiction, Anna Cora Mowatt's *The Mimic Life* is excellent for life upon the stage during the middle years of the 1880s and, as its author herself declared, "taken from life.")

1. Eric Wollencott Barnes, *The Lady of Fashion, the Life and the Theatre of Anna Cora Mowatt* (New York: Charles Scribner's Sons, 1954), p. 52.

2. *Ibid.*, p. 55.

3. Henry Austin Clapp, *Reminiscences of a Dramatic Critic* (Boston & New York: Houghton and Mifflin, 1902), p. 432.

4. *Ibid.*, pp. 432–3.

5. Barnes, p. 86.

6. *Ibid.*, p. 89.

7. Descriptions of stage life can be found in a number of books written by actors of the period such as *Footlight Flashes* by William Davidge, and *Before the Footlights and Behind the Scenes* by Olive Logan; Barnes' biography; Mrs. Mowatt's autobiography, and her *Mimic Life.*

8. Jack A. Vaughn, *Early American Dramatists from the Beginnings to 1900* New York: Frederick Ungar, 1981).

9. James Rees, *The Dramatic Authors of America* (Philadelphia: G.B. Zieber, 1845), p. 102.

10. *Ibid.*, p. 102.

11. *Ibid.*, p. 103.

12. Montrose J. Moses and John Mason Brown, *American Theatre as Seen by Its Critics (1752 to 1934),* (New York: W.W. Norton, 1967), p. 69.

13. *Ibid.*, pp. 64–66.

14. Oral Sumner Coad & Edward Mims, Jr., *The American Stage,* vol. 14, *The Pageant of America* (New Haven: Yale University Press, 1929), p. 117.

15. Laurence Hutton, *Curiosities of the American Stage* (New York: Harper & Bros., 1891), p. 63.

16. *Ibid.*, p. 66.

17. *Ibid.*, p. 63.

18. Webster's New International Dictionary, 2d ed., unabridged, defines Swedenborgianism thusly: "One who holds the doctrines of the New Jerusalem Church as taught by Emanuel Swedenborg, 1688–1772, a Swedish philosopher and religious writer. Swedenborg claimed to have direct intercourse with the spiritual world, through the opening of his spiritual senses in 1745. He taught that the Lord Jesus Christ, as comprehending in himself all the fullness of the Godhead, is the one and only God, and that there is a spiritual or symbolic meaning to the scriptures, which he [Swedenborg] was able to reveal because he saw the correspondence between natural and spiritual things."

19. Arthur Hobson Quinn, *A History of American Drama — 2 Vols.* (New York: F.S. Crofts, 1943), V. I, p. 319.

20. Vaughn p. 88.

21. Bernard Hewitt, *Theatre U.S.A. 1668–1957* (New York: McGraw-Hill, 1959), p. 141.

22. Barnes, p. 176–77; also Anna Cora Mowatt, *Autobiography of an Actress* (Boston: Ticknor and Fields, 1854), p. 249.

23. Barnes, p. 177.

24. Olive Logan, *Before the Footlights and Behind the Scene* (Philadelphia: n.p. 1870), p. 62.

25. Hutton, *Curiosities*, p. 67.

26. Logan, pp. 63–4.

27. Barnes, p. 167.

28. Perhaps, as in Manchester, they "acted for free" at first and agreed to indemnify the theatre management against losses.

29. Vaughn, p. 83.

30. *Ibid.*, p. 83.

31. Coad, p. 117.

32. Barnes, p. 258.

33. Quinn, p. 312.

34. Howard Taubman, *The Making of the American Theatre* (New York: Coward McCann, 1965), p. 76.

35. Hutton, *Curiosities*, p. 64.

36. Garff B. Wilson, *300 Years of American Drama and Theatre from "Ye Bare and Ye Cubb" to "Hair"* (Englewood Cliffs: Prentice-Hall, 1973), p. 172.

37. *Ibid.*, p. 173.

38. Hutton, *Curiosities*, p. 71.

39. Hewitt, p. 141.

40. *Ibid.*, p. 141.

41. Hutton, *Curiosities*, p. 64.

42. *Ibid.*, p. 70.

Sophia Turner

(Note: Sources are not given for statements which are generally accepted. This is the first time that information about Sopia Turner has been gathered together in biographical form. Anyone interested in further material about the early theatre on the frontier is referred to the following books [for complete citations, see the Bibliography]: Carson, W., *The Theatre on the Frontier*; Ludlow, Noah, *Dramatic Life as I Found It* [this collection of memoirs was written when Ludlow was nearly 80, and he was unable to see to edit it. It is sometimes inaccurate and subject to his prejudices, but fascinating reading, nonetheless]; Smith, Sol, *The Theatrical Apprenticeship of Sol Smith*; and West, T.H., *The Theatre in Early Kentucky*.)

1. Noah Ludlow, *Dramatic Life as I Found It* (n.p., reprinted 1966), pp. 65–67.

2. Anonymous, *Pittsburgh in 1816* (Pittsburgh: n.p., n.d.), p. 52.

3. *Lexington Reporter*, 2/23/1811, quoted in Beryl Meek, *A Record of the Theatre in Lexington, Kentucky from 1799*-1850 (M.A. Thesis: Univ. of Iowa, 1930), p. 59.

4. T. Hill West, Jr., *The Theatre in Early Kentucky 1790*-1820 (Lexington: University Press of Kentucky, 1971), p. 53 quoting *Gazette*, 1/1/1811.

5. West, p. 51.

6. George C.D. Odell, *Annals of the New York State to 1888* (New York: reissued 1927–1942), Vol. 2, pp. 293–294.

7. *Ibid.*, V. 2, p. 299.

8. Franklin Graham, *Histrionic Montreal* (Montreal: John Lovell & Son, 1902), p. 28. Graham lists David Douglas as a member of this company, but it is unlikely, since he was one of the earliest pioneers of theatre in this country. More probably the actor in question is his son James (Jimmie) Douglas who was known to be associated with the Montreal Theatre. James Douglas went south with William and Sophia, and was, nominally, the manager. He drowned nine years later in the Wabash River near Vincennes, Indiana.

9. *Ibid.*, p. 28.

10. *Ibid.*, p. 28.

11. Thomas Allston Brown, *History of the American Stage* (New York: Burt Franklin, reissued 1969), p. 363.

12. Lucile Naff Clay, *The Lexington Theatre from 1800*-1840 (Lexington, : M.A. Thesis, Univ. of Kentucky, 1930), p. 12.

13. *Ibid.*, p. 12.

14. Meek, p. 62. Possibly because of the penurious ways of Usher — see West, p. 76.

15. Clay, p. 18; West, p. 63.

16. West, p. 61.

17. *Ibid.*, pp. 67–8.

18. *Gazette*, 5/1/1812, quoted in: Sarah Killikelly, *The History of Pittsburgh, Its Rise and Fall* (Pittsburgh: B.C. & Gordon Montgomery, 1906), p. 529.

19. Killikelly, p. 529.

20. *Gazette*, 11/18/1813 quoted by Killikelly, p. 529.

21. *Pittsburgh Mercury*, 9/30/1813; this play was also the most popular in Lexington, being performed there nine times within a couple of years.

22. Page 2 of Western Pennsylvania Historical Society notes on early theatre in Pittsburgh.

23. West, pp. 99–101.

24. *Ibid.*, p. 101.

25. *Ibid.*, p. 101.

26. Ralph Leslie Rusk, *The Literature of the Middle Western Frontier* (New York: Frederick Ungar, 1925, 1953), Vol. I, 365–370, 440–443; West, pp. 99–101.

27. West, p. 104.

28. *Ibid.*, p. 107.

29. Ludlow, p. 116.

30. Rusk, Vol. 1, pp. 368–370. Turner brought suit against Noble Luke Usher, and advertised the double-dealing in the local papers. It was not his first run-in with Usher. See note 14.

31. Lewis F. Thomas, ed., Drawn and Lithographed by J.C. Wild, *The Valley of the Mississippi* (St. Louis: J.C. Wild, Chambers & Knapp, Printers, 1841), p. 24.

32. West, p. 52.

33. William G.B. Carson, *The Theatre on the Frontier, Early Years on the St. Louis Stage* (Chicago: Univ. of Chicago, 1932), p. 23.

34. *Ibid.*, p. 39.

35. West, p. 150.

36. Odell, V. III, p. 256.

37. *Ibid.*, V. III, pp. 369–370.

38. *Ibid.*, V. III, p. 361.

39. Francis Wemyss, *Wemyss' Chronology of the American Stage from 1752–1852* (New York: Benj. Blom, reissued 1968). Wemyss says that "she was on the stage in Philadelphia for a number of years," but there is no other evidence of this.

40. *Lexington Reporter*, 2/23/1811, quoted by Meek, p. 59.

Charlotte Cushman

(Note: Sources are not given for statements which are generally accepted. Anyone interested in further material about Charlotte Cushman is referred to the following books [for complete citations, see the Bibliography]: Stebbins, E., *Charlotte Cushman*; Faber, D., *Love and Rivalry*; Clement, C., *Charlotte Cushman.*)

1. William Winter, *Shadows of the Stage*, 1st Series. (New York: Macmillan, 1896), p. 206.

2. Garff B. Wilson, *300 Years of American Drama and Theatre from "Ye Bare and Ye Cubb" to "Hair,"* (Englewood Cliffs, N.J.: Prentice-Hall, 1973), pp. 95–98.

3. William Winter, *Other Days, Being Chronicles and Memories of the Stage,* (New York: Moffatt Yard, 1908), p. 153.

4. Emma Stebbins, *Charlotte Cushman, Her Letters and Memories of Her Life,* (Boston: Houghton, Osgood & Co., the Riverside Press, Cambridge, 1878), pp. 7–9; and Joseph Leach, *Bright Particular Sister* (New Haven: Yale University Press, 1970), pp. 1–3.

5. Stebbins, pp. 1–7.

6. Dorothy Faber, *Love and Rivalry: Three Exceptional Pairs of Sisters,* (New York: The Viking Press, 1983), p. 67.

7. Garff B. Wilson, *A History of American Acting,* (Bloomington & London: Indiana University Press, 1966), p. 49.

8. Gamaliel Bradford, *Biography and the Human Heart,* (Boston and New York: Houghton Mifflin, 1932), p. 112.

9. Lewis Clinton Strang, *Players and Plays of the Last Quarter Century,*

2 vols. (Boston: L.C. Page, 1902), Vol. 1, p. 99; and William Winter, *Shadows of the Stage,* 2d Series (Boston: Joseph Knight Co., 1893), p. 121.

10. Strang, Vol. I, p. 99–100.

11. Leach, pp. 37–45.

12. James H. Dormon Jr., *Theatre in the Ante-Bellum South* (Chapel Hill: University of North Carolina Press, 1967), p. 283; and Henry Pitt Phelps, *Players of a Century: A Record of the Albany Stage* (Albany: n.p. 1880), p. 200.

13. Faber, p. 80.

14. Clara Erskine Clement, *Charlotte Cushman* (American Actor Series), ed. by Lawrence Hutton (Boston: James R. Osgood, 1882), pp. 5–6.

15. Stebbins, pp. 25–27.

16. Clement, p. 8. The salary was to be $25 per week the first year and a $10 per week raise in each of the next two years. Hamblin kept $5 per week to pay for the wardrobe. During most of the 18th and 19th centuries, it was customary for actors to provide their own costumes which they did with wildly varying and frequently inappropriate results.

17. Phelps, p. 203.

18. Wilson, *History of American Acting,* p. 48.

19. Leach, p. 67.

20. Faber, p. 84.

21. Daniel Frohman, *Daniel Frohman Presents, An Autobiography* (New York: Claude Kendall and Willoughby Sharp, 1935), p. 17.

22. Joseph Norton Ireland, *Records of the New York Stage from 1750–1860,* 2 vols (n.p. 1866–67, reissued New York: Benjamin Blom, 1966), p. 216.

23. Leach quoting Wemyss, p. 70.

24. "Doats" — to be foolish or weak-minded especially because of old age.

25. Stebbins, pp. 147–152.

26. Legend has it that Otto Brahm who was appearing in *Guy Mannering* that evening was so stricken by the apparition of Charlotte Cushman as Meg that he was unable to continue his performance. However, Brahm was not in the cast the night and did not perform opposite Cushman in the play until long after her fame in the role would have made surprise unlikely.

27. Strang, Vol. I, p. 68.

28. Ireland, p. 271. *The Genoese,* also titled *The Bride of Genoa,* was by Epes Sargent.

29. Olive Logan, *The Mimic World* (Philadelphia: n.p., 1871), pp. 484–486.

30. Oral Sumner Coad & Edward Mims, Jr., *The American Stage,* Vol. 14 of *The Pageant of America* (New Haven: Yale University Press, 1929), p. 107.

31. Clement, p. 39.

32. Strang, Vol. I, p. 107. "Then she acted Lady Macbeth to the Macbeth of Edwin Forrest so successfully that after that night the two were never again friends." Laurence Barrett, *Charlotte Cushman: A Lecture, with an Appendix Containing a Letter from Joseph N. Ireland* (New York: The Dunlap Society,

1889), p. 19, suggests that Forrest threw up his engagement (quit performing in that role for that theatre) because her reception was so good, although this was later attributed to his anger at Macready's "machinations."

33. Winter, *Shadows*, 1st Series, pp. 209–210.

34. Josephine Clifton, an American, appeared at the Drury Lane in 1835, but Noah Ludlow in *Dramatic Life as I Found It* (n.p., reprinted 1966), p. 497, says "Her success as an actress was the result of careful training and an imposing personal appearance combined with fair average talents, for she possessed little of the true fire of genius."

35. Eleanor Ruggles, *The Prince of Players, Edwin Booth*, (New York: W.W. Norton & Co., Inc., 1953), p. 116.

36. John Rankin Towse, *Sixty Years of the Theatre*, (New York: Funk & Wagnalls, 1916), pp. 198–99.

37. Winter, *Other Days*, p. 158.

38. Ruggles, pp. 115–16.

39. Stanley Kimmel, *The Mad Booths of Maryland*, (Indianapolis: Bobbs-Merrill, 1940), p. 174.

40. William Winter, *Vagrant Memories, Being Further Recollections of Other Days* (New York; Geo. H. Doran, 1915), p. 69; and Joseph Jefferson, *An Autobiography* (n.p.: Century, 1890), p. 307; and Ludlow, p. 698.

41. Winter, *Shadows*, 2d Series, p. 132.

42. Henry Austin Clapp, *Reminiscences of a Dramatic Critic* (Boston & New York: Houghton & Mifflin, 1902), pp. 86–92.

43. Laurence Hutton, *Curiosities of the American Stage*, (New York: Harper & Bros., 1891), p. 322.

44. Helen Krick Chinoy, ed. and Linda Walsh Jenkins, ed., *Women in American Theatre Careers, Images, Movements: An Illustrated Anthology and Sourcebook*, (New York: Crown Publications, 1981), p. 78.

45. *Ibid.*, and Ruggles, p. 115.

46. Sheridan Knowles, Letter reprinted in the *Spirit of the Times*, (New York: n.p., July 4, 1846).

47. *Ibid.*

48. Winter, *Other Days*, p. 154.

49. Benjamin McArthur, *Actors & American Culture 1880–1920*, (Phildelphia: Temple University Press, 1984), p. 41.

50. Chinoy & Jenkins, p. 80.

51. Francis Courtney Wemyss, *Chronology of the American Stage*, (New York: n.p., 1852; reissued New York: Benjamin Blom, 1967), p. 41.

52. Bradford, p. 111.

53. Anesthesia, though suggested by Humphrey Davy in 1800, was not in general use until the mid to late 19th century. In 1842 a patient under the influence of ether was operated on, and certain studies were made during the American Civil War, but it was still a chancy procedure in 1869 when Charlotte Cushman was operated on.

54. The cause of Susan's death on May 12, 1859 has never been satisfactorily explained.

55. Winter, *Brief Chronicles*, p. 67.

56. Mary Caroline Crawford, *The Romance of the American Theatre*, (Boston: Little, Brown & Co., 1913).

57. Winter, *Other Days*, p. 167.

58. Henry P. Goddard, "Some Actresses I Have Known," *The Theatre Magazine*, VI (August, 1906), p. 206, cited in Wilson, *History*, p. 51.

59. Ruggles, p. 235.

60. Wilson, *History*, p. 51.

61. Logan, p. 284.

62. Winter, *Shadows*, 2nd Series, p. 131.

Laura Keene

(Note: Sources are not given for statements which are generally accepted. Anyone interested in further material about Laura Keene is referred to the following books [for complete citations, see the Bibliography]: Creahan, J., *The Life of Laura Keene*; there are numerous books on the life of Abraham Lincoln and his tragic assassination, most of which give some account of Laura Keene's part in that event.)

1. During his flight South, Booth stopped at the home of Dr. Mudd who set the actor's broken leg. Despite the fact that Mudd's complicity in the assassination was never proved, and, in fact, Mudd vehemently denied it, the doctor was sentenced to life imprisonment. His sentence was eventually commuted because of his services at the prison during an epidemic. Nonetheless, the shameful treatment the doctor received, gave rise to the expression "Your name is Mudd" for someone caught up in unwelcome notoriety.

2. Lloyd Lewis, *Myths After Lincoln* (New York: The Press of the Readers Club, 1941; first published by Harcourt Brace, 1929), p. 157. Edwin Booth was chased down alleyways by irate audience members after word of his brother's muderous actions became public. Edwin narrowly escaped with his life.

3. Boston Corbett, the sergeant who claimed responsibility for the killing of J.W. Booth. There was much controversy over this, since Corbett carried a revolver, and some authorities feel that Booth had to have been killed by a rifle. Corbett later sold his pistols, and eventully disappeared out West.

4. Lewis, p. 157; Olive Logan, *Before the Footlights and Behind the Scene* (Philadelphia: n.p., 1870), pp. 255–6.

5. Jim Bishop, *The Day Lincoln Was Shot* (New York: Harper, 1955), p. 131.

6. Mary Todd Lincoln gradually lost her grip on reality in the years after her husband's death, and she was not alone. There is a strong tradition of tragedy associated with Lincoln's assassination. Col. Rapp, who attended the theatre that night with the Lincolns, later married and murdered Clara Harris

who was also part of the group that evening. Clara Harris Rapp had also suffered from schizophrenia ever since April, 1865.

7. General Ulysses S. Grant attended another attraction in Washington, D.C., that evening, thus avoiding Booth's bullets. Later, his detractors would hint that he had advance warning to avoid Ford's Theatre. He went on to become as bad a president as he had been a good general.

8. Booth evaded capture for a number of days, but he was eventually run to ground in a barn where he was killed. There were numerous discrepancies concerning his death, and for years there were rumors that the body of the man killed that day was not that of John Wilkes Booth. His diary was recovered, but either before his death, or before it was released to the public, the pages relating to the days directly preceding the assassination were removed. There were other rumors of a larger conspiracy involving government officials, and "moneymen" who financed the whole plot.

9. William Winter, *Vagrant Memories, Being Further Recollections of Other Days* (New York: Geo. H. Doran, 1915), p. 55.

10. *Ibid.*, p. 49; Her name may also have been Mary Moss. Authorities are about evenly divided on the question. Creahan, Winter, and a variety of biographical sources including *Webster's Biographical Dictionary; Who Was Who in American History; The Dictionary of American Biography; Who Was Who in American History — Arts and Letters:* and the *National Cyclopedia of American Biography,* all say her family name was Lee or "unknown." On the other hand, an equal number of sources maintain that she was Mary Moss, of a respectable London family, that she frequented the studio of Turner, the painter, as a child, and that her aunt, Mrs. Yates, was an actress in London. Proponents of this point of view include Garff B. Wilson writing in *Notable American Women; Webster's American Biographies; The New Encyclopaedia Britannica Micropedia;* and *The World Scope Encyclopedia* which also includes the statement, ". . . Laura Keene being the stage name given to her by Charles Reade." Reade, of course, is the well-known author of *The Cloister and the Hearth.* See also Notes 16 & 27.

11. Joseph Ireland, cited by Winter, *Vagrant Memories,* p. 49.

12. John Creahan, cited by Winter, *Vagrant Memories,* p. 49.

13. Winter, *Vagrant Memories,* p. 49.

14. Creahan, cited by Winter, *Vagrant Memories,* p. 49, but Arthur Hornblow, *A History of the Theatre in America* (New York: Benj. Blom, reissued 1965), pp. 208-9, says that Rachel occupied Laura Keene's theatre in America immediately before she took over the building, so it is possible that Laura Keene saw her perform in America.

15. Winter, *Vagrant Memories* p. 49.

16. Winter goes to great lengths to prove that Madame Vestris never produced this play.

17. Hornblow, p. 186.

18. Stanley Kimmel, *The Mad Booths of Maryland* (New York, Indianapolis: Bobbs-Merrill, 1940), pp. 108-9; Eleanor Ruggles, *The Prince of Players* (New York: W.W. Norton, 1953), p. 69.

19. Winter, *Vagrant Memories,* p. 58; Kimmel also says that Taylor was imprisoned before Keene went on the stage and that that was why she took up acting. He also says that her cross-country trek was, at least in part, to search for Taylor and that she was accompanied by John Lutz.

20. Joseph Jefferson, *An Autobiography* (New York: Century, 1890), p. 146.

21. Winter, *Vagrant Memories,* p. 58.

22. Mordaunt, quoted in Garff B. Wilson, *A History of American Acting* (Bloomington & London: Indiana University Press, 1966), p. 120.

23. Winters, *Vagrant Memories,* p. 51.

24. Glenn Hughes, *History of the American Theatre 1700–1951* (New York: Samuel French, 1951), pp. 179–80.

25. Winter, *Vagrant Memories,* p. 52.

26. Ruggles, p. 69.

27. Kimmel, p. 116; he also says that Taylor was in prison for life, but this is probably not true. *The World Scope Encyclopedia* gives her husband's name as Henry Wellington Taylor, the only authority for this name I could find.

28. William Winter, *Brief Chronicles* (New York: B. Franklin, 1970), pp. 178–81; Joseph Norton Ireland, *Records of the New York Stage from 1750–1860* (New York: Benj. Blom, reissued 1966), Vol. 2, p. 649; Ruggles and others also say that when the tour was ended, Booth and Keene and the other actors stopped in Hawaii to play long enough to get money for passage to the States, implying that the tour was less than successful. Laura Keene, however, did not stay to perform with them, but went on ahead, notified a California manager that Booth was coming, and would likely need a job, and then went on to New York to open her theatre. Why Laura Keene had the money to do this when the others did not, is not clear.

29. Hughes, p. 183–4.

30. Hornblow, p. 185.

31. Catherine Mary Reignolds-Winslow, *Yesterdays with Actors* (Boston: Cupples & Hurd, 1887), pp. 71–2.

32. Winters, *Vagrant Memories* pp. 46–7.

33. Archie Binns, *Mrs. Fiske and the American Theatre* (New York: Crown, 1955), p. 140.

34. John Creahan, *The Life of Laura Keene* (Philadelphia: Rodgers, 1897), p. 128; of course, there is no record of Laura Keene ever having had a theatre in California.

35. Jefferson, p. 139.

36. *Ibid.,* pp. 140–44.

37. *Ibid.,* pp. 150–1.

38. *Ibid.,* p. 150.

39. *Ibid.,* p. 147.

40. Crehan, pp. 131–2.

41. W. Emerson Reck, *A. Lincoln: His Last 24 Hours* (Jefferson, N.C.: McFarland, 1987), p. 118.

42. *Ibid.*, p. 123; Bishop, p. 217.

43. Reck, p. 123.

44. Bishop, p. 267-8; Lewis, pp. 156-7; Kimmel, p. 263.

45. Reck, pp. 116-7.

46. Lewis, p. 157; some authorities suggest that the arrest was made in Harrisburg, Pa., *the following day*, April 15, 1865, which is unlikely, to say the least.

47. Winter, *Brief Chronicles*, p. 180.

48. Reck, p. 92.

49. Montrose J. Moses, *The American Dramatist* (Boston: n.p., 1911) p. 158.

50. William Winter, *The Life and Art of Joseph Jefferson* (New York: Macmillan, 1894), pp. 242-3.

51. Creahan, p. 123.

52. Reck, p. 91.

Mrs. John Drew

(Note: Sources are not given for statements which are generally accepted. Anyone interested in further material about Mrs. John Drew is referred to the following books [for complete citations, see the Bibliography]: Drew, Mrs. J., *An Autobiographical Sketch*; all three of Mrs. Drew's Barrymore grandchildren wrote autobiographies which give details about their lives, but less about their grandmother. Barrymore, L., *We Barrymores*; Barrymore, J., *Confessions of an Actor*; Barrymore, E., *Memories*; James Kotsilibas-Davis wrote two books on the Barrymore dynasty which can be recommended [they deal with the Drews as well]: *Good Times, Great Times; The Barrymores, The Royal Family*.)

1. George Kaufman & Edna Ferber, *The Royal Family* (1927). This play is supposed to be based on the Drew-Barrymore clan, and Ethel Barrymore was actually offered the opportunity to play the character based on her in the initial production. She refused indignantly.

2. Oral Sumner Coad & Edward Mims, Jr., *The American Stage*, Vol. 14, *The Pageant of America* (New Haven: Yale Univ. Press, 1929), p. 97.

3. Mrs. John Drew, *An Autobiographical Sketch of Mrs. John Drew* (New York: Charles Scribner's Sons, 1899), pp. 13-17.

4. Coad, p. 97.

5. Mrs. Drew, pp. 29-30.

6. *Ibid.*, pp. 34-37.

7. James Kotsilibas-Davis, *Good Times, Great Times, The Odyssey of Maurice Barrymore* (Garden City, N.Y.: Doubleday, 1977), p. 88.

8. Mrs. Drew, pp. 65-66.

9. Montrose J. Moses, *Famous Actor-Families in America* (New York: Benj. Blom, 1906), p. 173.

10. John Kobler, *Damned in Paradise, The Life of John Barrymore* (New York: Atheneum, 1977), p. 9.

11. Joseph Jefferson, *An Autobiography* (New York: Century, 1890), p. 306.

12. Moses, p. 173.

13. Ethel Barrymore, *Memories, An Autobiography* (New York: Harper & Bros., 1955), p. 4.

14. Kotsilibas-Davis, p. 102.

15. Coad, p. 97.

16. Moses, p. 177.

17. Otis Skinner, quoted in Jack Poggi, *Theater in America* (Ithaca, N.Y.: Cornell University Press, 1968), p. 251.

18. Clara Morris, "Where I First Met Ellen Terry and Mrs. John Drew (A Dressing Room Reception)," *McClure's Magazine,* (1903: 22: 204-11, December), p. 210.

19. *Ibid.,* p. 210.

20. Augustus Thomas, *The Print of My Remembrancce* (New York: 1922), p. 130, quoted in Poggi, p. 252.

21. Coad, p. 198.

22. Mrs. Drew, pp. 141–142.

23. Glenn Hughes, *History of the American Theatre 1700 – 1951*), p. 210.

24. Moses, p. 180.

25. Frederick E. McKay, *Famous American Actors of Today* (New York: n.p. 1896), pp. 130–133.

26. Clara Morris, p. 210.

27. Kotsilibas-Davis, p. 103.

28. *Ibid.,* p. 102.

29. According to theatrical legend, when Ada Rehan was 17 and making her debut at the Arch Street Theatre, the printer made an error, transforming her from ADA CREHAN to ADA C. REHAN. Ever after that she was known as Ada Rehan. Mary Caroline Crawford, *The Romance of the American Theatre* (Boston: Little Brown, 1925), p. 374.

30. Barrymore, E. p. 8.

31. Jefferson, p. 297.

32. John Drew, *My Years on the Stage* (E.P. Dutton, 1922), pp. 1-5.

33. Kobler, pp. 19–20.

34. Barrymore, E., p. 5.

35. *Ibid.,* pp. 42–43.

36. Lionel Barrymore, *We Barrymores* (New York: Appleton-Century-Crofts, 1951), p. 84.

Fanny Kemble

(Note: Sources are not given for statements which are generally accepted. Anyone interested in further material about Fanny Kemble is referred to the following biographies [for complete citation see the Bibliography]: Armstrong, M., *Fanny Kemble, A Passionate Victorian;* Bobbe, D., *Fanny Kemble;* Driver, L. *Fanny Kemble;* Fitzgerald, P., *The Kembles;* Furnas, J., *Fanny Kemble, Leading Lady of the 19th Century Stage;* Pope-

Hennessy, Dame U., *Three Englishwomen in America;* Rushmore, R., *Fanny Kemble;* Wright, C., *Fanny Kemble and the Lovely Land.*)

1. Oral Sumner Coad and Edward Mims, Jr., *The American Stage* (New Haven: Yale Univ. Press, 1929), Vol. 14, *The Pageant of America* p. 102.

2. Ann Kemble later married a Mr. Hatton, came to America, wrote a play *Tammany,* about an Indian chief, and became involved in New York politics. Her husband became a famous instrument maker.

3. Sir Richard Arkwright invented a spinning frame, a carding machine, and a secret method of dyeing human hair. He also built the first cotton mills which have been called the beginning of the factory system.

4. Her brother, Vincent deCamp, was a "Bath Beau" (intimate of George IV), became an American actor, then an unsuccessful dairy farmer in Houston, Texas, where he died in 1839. See Carson, *Theatre on the Frontier* pp. 185-6.

5. Joseph Norton Ireland, *Records of the New York Stage from 1750-1860* (New York: Benj. Blom, 1966) Vol. 1. pp. 40-1.

6. Mary Caroline Crawford, *The Romance of the American Theatre* (Boston: Little, Brown, 1925), p. 239, quoting the *New York Mirror* of Sept. 22, 1832.

7. Margaret Davis Cate, "Mistakes in Fanny Kemble's Georgia Journal" (*Georgia Historical Quarterly*, Vol. XLIV #1, March 1960), p. 3.

8. *Ibid.*, p. 3.

9. Frances Anne Kemble, *Journal of a Residence on a Georgia Plantation 1838-1839*, edited with an Introduction by John A. Scott (Athens: Univ. of Georgia Press, 1984), pp. 60-1.

10. *Ibid.*, p. 61.

11. *Ibid.*, p. 61.

12. *Ibid.*, p. 61.

13. *Ibid.*, p. 100.

14. *Ibid.*, p. 70.

15. *Ibid.*, p. 68.

16. *Ibid.*, p. 68.

17. *Ibid.*, p. 68.

18. Joseph Chamberlain Furnas, *Fanny Kemble, Leading Lady of the 19th Century Stage*, (New York: the Dial Press, 1982) p. 237.

19. Pierce Butler, "Mr. Butler's Statement" (Philadelphia: n.p., 1850), privately printed, p. 67.

20. William Davidge, *Footlight Flashes*, (New York: American News Co., 1866), p. 79.

21. *Ibid.*, p. 79.

22. Furnas, p. 308.

23. MacReady became involved in the Astor Place Riots in 1849 in which Edwin Forrest's supporters who (falsely) held MacReady responsible for Forrest's poor English reception, created disturbances during MacReady's production of *Macbeth.*

24. Henry Austin Clapp, *Reminiscences of a Dramatic Critic*, (Boston and New York: Houghton & Mifflin, 1902), p. 178.

25. Furnas, p. 353.

26. Furnas, p. 391–405 *passim.*

27. Furnas, pp. 362–3.

Minnie Maddern Fiske

(Note: Sources are not given for statements which are generally accepted. Anyone interested in further material about Minnie Maddern Fiske is referred to the following books [for complete citations, see the Bibliography]: Binns, A., *Mrs. Fiske & the American Stage* [the only full-fledged biography]; and Woollcott, A., *Mrs. Fiske, Her Views on the Stage.*)

1. (Franklin P. Adams, quoted in Archie Binns in collaboration with Olive Kooken,) *Mrs. Fiske and the American Stage* (New York: Crown, 1955), p. 227.

2. Binns, pp. 21–22.

3. Bernard Hewitt, *Theatre U.S.A. 1668–1957* (New York: McGraw-Hill, 1959), p. 302.

4. Lewis C. Strang, *Famous Actresses of the Day in America,* 1st series (Boston: L. C. Page & Co., 1899), pp. 66–7.

5. Helen Ormsbee, *Backstage with Actors* (New York: Thomas Y. Crowell, 1938), p. 198.

6. Hewitt, p. 256.

7. Glenn Hughes, *History of the American Theatre, 1700–1951* (New York: Samuel French, 1951), p. 318.

8. Oral Sumner Coad and Edward Mims, Jr., *The American Stage, The Pageant of America,* Vol. 14 (New Haven: Yale University Press, 1929), p. 308.

9. Lewis C. Strang, *Players and Plays of the Last Quarter Century* (Boston: L.C. Page & Co., 1902), p. 218.

10. Ethan Mordden, *The American Theatre* (New York: Oxford University Press, 1981), p. 29.

11. *Ibid.,* p. 29.

12. Garff B. Wilson, *A History of American Acting* (Bloomington and London: Indiana University Press, 1966), p. 235.

13. *Ibid.,* p. 235.

14. Ormsbee, p. 199.

15. Mordden, p. 29.

16. Garff B. Wilson, *300 Years of American Drama and Theatre from "Ye Bare and Ye Cubb" to "Hair"* (Englewood Cliffs: Prentice-Hall, 1973), p. 320.

17. Ormsbee, p. 199.

18. Wilson, *300* . . . , p. 321.

19. Binns, p. 151.

20. *Ibid.,* p. 166.

21. Amy Leslie, *Some Players: Personal Sketches* (Chicago & New York: Herbert S. Stone, 1899), p. 106.

22. Ormsbee, p. 202.

23. *Ibid.*, p. 202.

24. Binns, p. 191.

25. Sheldon was a product of George Pierce Baker's "Workshop 47" at Harvard.

26. Binns, p. 204.

27. Wilson, *300*... p. 321.

28. Binns, p. 213.

29. *Ibid.*, p. 251–2.

30. *Ibid.*, p. 394.

31. Ormsbee, p. 202.

32. Hughes, p. 263.

33. John Rankin Towse, *Sixty Years of the Theatre* (New York: Funk and Wagnalls Co., 1916), p. 411–13.

34. Leslie, p. 106.

35. Wilson, *300*..., p. 317, 321.

36. *Ibid.*, p. 319.

37. *Ibid.*, p. 318.

38. *Ibid.*, p. 318.

BIBLIOGRAPHY

Adams, Oscar Fay. "Susanna Haswell Rowson," *Christian Register* **17** (March 1913): pp. 296–299. (April 1913): p. 321.

Alpert, Hollis. *The Barrymores.* New York: The Dial Press, 1964.

Anderson, John. *The American Theatre.* New York: The Dial Press, 1938.

The Assassination and History of the Conspiracy. A Complete digest of the affair from its inception to its culmination, Sketches of the principal Characters, Reports of the Obsequies, etc. Cincinnati: J.R. Hawley, 1865.

Armstrong, Margaret. *Fanny Kemble, A Passionate Victorian.* New York: Macmillan, 1938.

Baldwin, Leland D. *Pittsburgh, The Story of a City.* Pittsburgh: University of Pittsburgh Press, 1938.

Barnes, Eric Wollencott. *The Lady of Fashion, The Life and the Theatre of Anna Cora Mowatt.* New York: Charles Scribner's Sons, 1954.

Barrymore, Diana. *Too Much Too Soon.* New York: Henry Holt, 1957.

Barrymore, Ethel. *Memories, An Autobiography.* New York: Harper & Bros., 1955.

Barrymore, John. *Confessions of an Actor.* New York: Benj. Blom, reprint 1971.

Barrymore, Lionel. *We Barrymores.* Westport, Conn.: Greenwood Press, reprint 1974.

Berquist, G. William. *Three Centuries of English & American Plays, A Checklist, England 1500–1800; U.S. 1714–1830.* New York: n.p. 1963.

Binns, Archie, in collaboration with Olive Kooken. *Mrs. Fiske and the American Stage.* New York: Crown, 1958.

Bishop, James Alonzo. *The Day Lincoln Was Shot.* New York: Harper, 1955.

Bobbe, Dorothie. *Fanny Kemble.* New York: Minton Black, 1931.

Bowen, Marjorie. *Peter Porcupine, A Study of William Cobbett, 1762–1835.* London, New York, Toronto: Longmans, Green, 1936.

Bradford, Gamaliel. *Biography and the Human Heart.* Boston, New York: Houghton Mifflin, 1932.

Brown, Thomas Allston. *History of the American Stage, a series of biographical sketches.* New York: 1870. New York: Burt Franklin, reprinted 1969.

Buckingham, Joseph T. *Personal Memoirs & Recollections of Editorial Life.* Boston: n.p. 1852, Vol. I.

Burge, James C. *Lines of Business, Casting Practice and Policy in the American*

Theatre 1752–1899. American University Studies, Series IX, History, Vol. 19. New York, Berne, Frankfurt am Main: Peter Lang, 1986.

Butler, Pierce. "Mr. Butler's Statement." Philadelphia: Privately printed, n.p., 1850.

Carson, William G.B. *Managers in Distress, the St. Louis Stage 1840–1844.* St. Louis: 1949. New York: 1965.

————. *The Theatre on the Frontier, The Early Years of the St. Louis Stage.* Chicago: University of Chicago Press, 1932. Reprinted, New York: Benj. Blom, 1965.

Cate, Margaret Davis. "Mistakes in Fanny Kemble's Georgia Journal." *Georgia Historical Quarterly,* Vol. XLIV #1 (March 1961).

Charvat, William. *The Profession of Authorship in America 1800–1870.* Ed. Matthew Bruccoli, Foreword by Howard Mumford Jones. Columbus, Ohio: Ohio State University Press, 1968.

————. *Literary Publishing in America 1790–1850.* Philadelphia: University of Pennsylvania Press, 1959.

Chinoy, Helen Krick, and Linda Walsh Jenkins, eds. *Women in American Theatre: Careers, Images, Movements. An Illustrated Anthology and Sourcebook.* New York: Crown, 1981.

Clapp, Henry Austin. *Reminiscences of a Dramatic Critic.* Boston & New York: Houghton & Mifflin, 1902.

Clapp, John Bouve, and Edwin Francis Edgett. *Players of the Present 1899–1901.* New York: Burt Franklin Research Series, n.d.

Clapp, W.W., Jr. *A Record of the Boston Stage.* Cambridge & Boston: J. Monroe, 1853.

Clark, Barrett H. *An Hour of American Drama.* Philadelphia: J.B. Lippincott, 1930.

Clay, Lucile Naff. *The Lexington Theatre from 1800 – 1840.* Lexington, KY.: M.A. Thesis, Univeristy of Kentucky, 1930.

Clement, Clara Erskine. *Charlotte Cushman.* Boston: James R. Osgood, 1882.

Cobbett, William (Peter Porcupine, pseud.). *A Kick for a Bite: a Review Upon Review; with a critical Essay on the works of Mrs. S. Rowson, in a letter to the Editor or Editors of the American Monthly Review.* Philadelphia: Thomas Bradford, 1795.

Coder, William D. *A History of the Philadelphia Theatre 1856–1878.* Philadelphia: doctoral dissertation, University of Pennsylvania, 1936.

Cole, G.D.H. *The Life of William Cobbett,* with a Chapter by F.E. Green. London: W. Collins & Sons, 1924/25.

Cone, Helen Gray, and Jeannette L. Gilder. *Pen-Portraits of Literary Women by Themselves and Others.* Vol. I. New York: Cassell, 1887.

Cottrell, John. *Anatomy of an Assassination, The Murder of Abraham Lincoln.* New York: Funk & Wagnalls, 1966.

Cowell, Joe. *Thirty Years Passed Among the Actors and Actresses of England and America.* New York: n.p. 1844.

Coad, Oral Sumner, and Edward Mims, Jr. *The American Stage,* Vol. 14 "The Pageant of America." New Haven: Yale University Press, 1929.

Crawford, Mary Caroline. *The Romance of the American Theatre.* Boston: Little, Brown, 1913. Rev. ed. 1925.

Creahan, John. *The Life of Laura Keene.* Philadelphia: Rodgers Publ., 1897.

Dale, Alan. *Familiar Chats with the Queens of the Stage.* New York: G.W. Dillingham, 1890.

Daly, Charles Patrick. *The First Theatre in America, An Inquiry.* Port Washington, N.Y.: Kennikat Press, 1968. orig. publ. 1896 by the Dunlap Society.

Davidge, William. *Footlight Flashes by Wm. Davidge, Comedian.* American News, 1866.

Dexter, Elizabeth Anthony. *Colonial Women of Affairs: A Study of Women in Business and the Professions in America before 1776.* Boston: Hougton, Mifflin, 1924.

Dithmar, Edward Augustus. *John Drew.* New York: Frederick A. Stokes, 1900. 2nd Ed.

Dormon, James H., Jr. *Theatre in the Ante-Bellum South 1815-1816.* Chapel Hill: University of North Carolina Press, 1967.

Doty, Gresdna Ann. *The Career of Mrs. Anne Brunton Merry in the American Theatre.* Baton Rouge: Louisiana State University Press, 1971.

Downer, Alan S., ed. *The Memoir of John Durang, American Actor 1785-1816.* Pittsburgh: Published for the Historical Society of York County and for the American Society of Theatre Research by the University of Pittsburgh Press, 1966.

Drew, John. *My Years on the Stage.* New York: E.P. Dutton, 1922.

Drew, Mrs. John (Louisa Lane). *An Autobiographical Sketch of Mrs. John Drew.* New York: Charles Scribner's Sons, 1899.

Driver, Leota S. *Fanny Kemble.* Chapel Hill: University of North Carolina Press, 1933.

Dunlap, William A. *History of the American Theatre.* 2 vols. New York: n.p., 1832. London: n.p., 1833. Reprinted New York: Burt Franklin, 1963.

Eisenschiml, Otto. *In the Shadow of Lincoln's Death.* New York: Wilfred Funk, 1940.

Faber, Dorothy. *Love and Rivalry, Three Exceptional Pairs of Sisters.* New York: The Viking Press, 1983.

Ferber, Edna, and George Kaufman. *The Royal Family.* Produced 1927.

Fiske, Minnie Maddern. *A Light from St. Agnes.* From: *One Act Plays for Stage and Study.* 9th Series. Preface by Garrett H. Leverton. New York, Los Angeles, London, Toronto: Samuel French, 1938.

Fitzgerald, Percy Hetherington. *The Kembles: An Account of the Kemble Family Including the Lives of Mrs. Siddons, and Her Brother John Philip Kemble.* London: Tinsley Bros., 1871.

Ford, Thomas. *The Actor; or, A Peep Behind the Curtain by a Supernumerary, Being Passages in the Lives of J.B. Booth and His Contemporaries.* New York: Wm. H. Graham, 1846.

Fowler, Gene. *Good Night, Sweet Prince.* Philadelphia: The Blakeston Co., 1945.

Fowler, Robert H. *Album of the Lincoln Murder: Illustrating How It Was Planned, Committed, & Avenged.* Civil War Times. Harrisburg, PA: Historical Times, Inc., Stackpole Books, 1965.

Fraser, Antonia. *The Weaker Vessel.* New York: Vintage, 1985.

Frohman, Daniel. *Daniel Frohman Presents, an Autobiography.* New York: Claude Kendall & Willoughby Sharp, 1935.

Furnas, Joseph Chamberlain. *Fanny Kemble, Leading Lady of the 19th Century Stage.* New York: The Dial Press, 1982.

Fyles, Franklin. *Theatre and Its People.* New York: Doubleday, Page, 1900.

Gergenheimer, A.F. "Early History of the Philadelphia Stage," *Pennsylvania History,* IX (1942), pp. 233–241.

Goodale, Katharine (Kitty Moloney). *Behind the Scenes with Edwin Booth, with a Foreword by Mrs. Fiske.* Boston, New York: Houghton Mifflin, 1931.

Graham, Franklin. *Histrionic Montreal.* Montreal: John Lovell & Sons, 1902.

Grimstead, David. *Melodrama Unveiled, American Theatre and Culture 1800–1850.* Chicago: University of Chicago Press, 1968.

Griswold, Rufus Wilmot. *Female Poets of America.* Philadelphia: Carey & Hart, 1843.

Hahn, Emily. *Once Upon a Pedestal.* New York: Thomas Y. Crowell, 1974.

Halliburton, William, Esq. *Effects of the Stage on the Manners of a People: and the Propriety of Encouraging and Establishing a Virtuous Theatre, by a Bostonian.* Boston: Printed by Young & Ethrege, 1792.

Hamm, Margherita Arlina. *Eminent Actors in Their Homes, Personal Descriptions and Interviews.* New York: James Pott, 1902.

Hapgood, Norman. *The Stage in America 1897–1900.* New York: n.p., 1901.

Harland, Marion. "Personal Recollections of a Christian Actress." *Our Continent,* I (March 15, 1882), pp. 73–74.

Hewitt, Bernard. *Theatre U.S.A. 1668–1957.* New York: McGraw-Hill, 1959.

Hodge, Francis. *Yankee Theatre, The Image of America on the Stage 1825–1850.* Austin: University of Texas Press, 1964.

Hornblow, Arthur. *A History of the Theatre in America.* 2 Vols. Philadelphia: J.B. Lippincott, 1919. Reissued: New York: Benj. Blom, 1965.

Howay, F.W. "A Short Account of Robert Haswell." *Washington Historical Quarterly* 24 (1933), pp. 83–90.

Hughes, Glenn. *History of the American Theatre 1700–1951.* New York: Samuel French, 1951.

Hutton, Laurence. *Curiosities of the American Stage.* New York: Harper & Bros. 1891.

————. *Actors & Actresses of Great Britain and the U.S.A.* n.p., 1886.

Ireland, Joseph Norton. *Fifty Years of a Playgoers Journal 1798–1848.* New York: n.p., 1860.

————. *Records of the New York Stage from 1750–1860.* 2 Vols. n.p., 1866–67. Reissued: New York: Benj. Blom, 1966.

Jefferson, Joseph. *An Autobiography.* New York: Century, 1890.

James, Edward T., ed. *Notable American Women 1607–1950.* Cambridge: Belknap Press of Harvard University Press, 1971.

James, Reese Davis. *Cradle of Culture 1800–1810; The Philadelphia Stage.* Philadelphia: University of Pennsylvania Press, 1957.

_____. *Old Drury of Philadelphia, A History of the Philadephia Stage 1800–1835.* (including a reprint of William Wood's Diary). Philadelphia: University of Pennsylvania Press, 1932.

Kable, William S. *Three American Novels* (including) *Charlotte: A Tale of Truth by Susannah Haswell Rowson.* Introduction by Wm. S. Kable. Columbus, Ohio: Charles E. Merrill, 1970.

Kemble, Frances Anne. *Journal of a Residence in America (Journal of a Residence on a Georgia Plantation).* Edited with an Introduction by John A. Scott. Athens: Brown Thrasher Books, University of Georgia Press, 1984.

_____. *Records of a Girlhood.* New York: Henry Holt, 1889.

_____. *Journal of Frances Anne Butler.* 2 Vols. Philadelphia: Carey, Lea, & Blanchard, 1835.

_____. *Further Records.* New York: Henry Holt, 1891.

_____. *Records of a Later Life.* New York: Henry Holt, 1882.

Killikelly, Sarah. *The History of Pittsburgh, Its Rise and Fall.* Pittsburgh: B.C. & Gordon Montgomery Co. 1906.

Kimmel, Stanley, *The Mad Booths of Maryland.* Indianapolis: Bobbs-Merrill, 1940.

Kirk, Clara M., and Rudolph Kirk. "Introduction," *Charlotte Temple: A Tale of Truth.* Twayne's United States Classics Series. New York: Twayne Publishers, 1964.

Kobler, John. *Damned in Paradise. The Life of John Barrymore.* New York: Atheneum, 1977.

Kotsilibas-Davis, James. *The Barrymores, The Royal Family in Hollywood.* New York: Crown Publishers, 1981.

_____. *Great Times Good Times, The Odyssey of Maurice Barrymore.* Garden City, N.Y.: Doubleday, 1977.

Kunhardt, Dorothy Meserve & Philip B., Jr. *Twenty Days.* Foreword by Bruce Catton. New York: Harper & Row, 1965.

Leach, Joseph. *Bright Particular Sister.* New Haven: Yale University Press, 1970.

Leslie, Amy. *Some Players: Personal Sketches.* Chicago & New York: Herbert S. Stone, 1899.

Lewis, Lloyd. *Myths After Lincoln.* New York: Harcourt, Brace, 1929.

Logan, Olive. *Apropos of Women and Theatre.* Charleston: n.p., 1869.

_____. *Before the Footlights and Behind the Scene.* Philadelphia: n.p., 1870.

_____. *The Mimic World.* Philadelphia: n.p., 1871.

Ludlow, Noah. *Dramatic Life as I Found It.* n.d., n.p. Reissued 1966.

McArthur, Benjamin. *Actors and American Culture 1880–1920.* Philadelphia: Temple University Press, 1984.

McKay, Frederick Edward, and Charles E.L. Wingate. *Famous American Actors of Today.* (Mrs. John Drew by T. Allston Brown.) New York: Thomas Y. Crowell, 1896.

Maeder, Clara Fisher. *Autobiography of Clara Fisher,* ed. by Douglas Taylor. New York: Dunlap Society Publications M.S. #3, 1897.

Malone, Dumas. *Dictionary of American Biography.* New York: Charles Scribner's Sons, 1932-33.

Malpede, Karen. *Women in the Theatre, Compassion & Hope.* Edited with an Introduction and Notes by Karen Malpede. New York: Drama Books Publishers., 1983.

Marcossan, Isaac F., and Daniel Frohman. *Charles Frohman, Manager & Man.* New York & London: Harper & Bros., 1916.

Marshall, Thomas F. *A History of the Philadelphia Theatre for 1878-1879, and a Checklist of Plays 1878-1890.* Westminster, Maryland: n.p., 1944.

Mates, Julian. *The American Musical Stage Before 1800.* New Brunswick: Rutgers University Press, 1962.

Matthews, Brander. *A Book About the Theatre.* New York: n.p., 1916.

_____. *Books and Playbooks.* London: n.p., 1895.

_____. *The Development of the Drama.* New York: n.p., 1903.

_____. "Drama in the 18th Century." *Sewanee Review* **XI** (1903), I.

_____. *Rip Van Winkle Goes to the Play.* New York: n.p., 1926.

_____. *These Many Years.* New York: n.p., 1917.

Mayorga, Margaret G. *A Short History of the American Drama.* New York: Dodd, Mead, 1932, 1934.

Mease, James, M.D. *The Picture of Philadelphia.* Philadelphia: B. & T. Kite, 1811.

Meek, Beryl. *A Record of the Theatre in Lexington, Kentucky from 1799-1850.* M.A. Thesis, University of Iowa, 1930.

Moody, Richard. *America Takes the Stage.* Bloomington: Indiana University Press, 1955.

_____. *Dramas from the American Theatre 1762-1909.* Edited, with an Introductory Essay by Richard Moody. Cleveland: World Publishing, 1966.

Mordden, Ethan. *The American Theatre.* New York: Oxford University Press, 1981.

Morris, Clara. "Where I First Met Ellen Terry and Mrs. John Drew [A Dressing Room Reception]" *McClure's Magazine* 1903: 22:204-211, December.

Morris, Lloyd. *Curtain Times: The Story of American Theatre.* New York: 1953.

Moses, Montrose J. *The American Dramatist.* Boston: n.p., 1911. Rev. ed., 1925.

_____. *Famous Actor-Families in America.* New York: n.p., 1906. Reissued Benj. Blom.

Moses, Montrose J., and John Mason Brown. *The American Theatre as Seen by Its Critics (1752-1934).* New York: W.W. Norton, 1934.

Mowatt, Anna Cora. *Autobiography of an Actress.* Boston: Ticknor & Fields, 1854.

_____. *Autobiography of an Actress, or, Eight Years on the Stage.* Boston: n.p., 1854.

_____. *Mimic Life: or, Before and Behind the Curtain.* Boston: Ticknor and Fields, 1856.

Murdoch, James E. *The Stage or Recollections of Actors and Acting from an Experience of Fifty Years.* Philadelphia: n.p., 1880. Reissued New York: Benj. Blom, 1969.

Nason, Elias, M.A. *A Memoir of Mrs. Susanna Rowson.* Albany: Joel Munsell, 1870. Originall prepared as a lecture for the New York Historical and Genealogical Society, 1859.

The National Cyclopedia of American Biography, Vol. 8. Ann Arbor: University Microfilms, 1967. Orig. publ. James T. White & Co., 1898.

New York Times. "Charlotte Temple's Tomb," by Mary A. Taft. 7/9/1905.

Northall, William Knight. *Before and Behind the Curtain, or Fifty Years Observations.* New York: n.p., 1851.

Oberholtzer, E.P. *Literary History of Philadelphia.* Philadelphia: n.p., 1906.

Odell, George C.D. *Annals of the New York Stage* Vols. 1–13 (to 1888.) New York: n.p., 1927–1942.

Ornsbee, Helen. *Backstage with Actors.* New York: Thomas Y. Crowell, 1938.

Papavashivily, Helen Waite. *All The Happy Endings: A Study of the Domestic Novel in America, the Women Who Wrote It, the Women Who Read It, in the Nineteenth Century.* New York: Harper & Bros., 1956.

Parker, John, comp. and ed. *Who's Who in the Theatre, A Biographical record of the Contemporary Stage.* 10th Edition, revised. New York, Chicago: Pitman Publishing, 1947.

Parker, Patricia L. *Susanna Rowson.* Boston: Twayne Publ., 1981.

Paul, Howard. *The Stage and Its Stars, Past and Present.* New York: n.p., 1895.

Phelps, Henry Pitt. *Players of a Century: A Record of the Albany Stage.* Albany: n.p., 1880.

_____. *Addenda to Players of a Century.* Albany: n.p. 1889.

Pittsburgh in 1866. Pittsburgh: n.p., n.d.

Plumb, Harriet Pixley. *Charlotte Temple, A Historical Drama, in Three Acts with a Prologue.* Chicago & London: Publishers Printing Co., T. Fisher Unwin, 1899.

Poggi, Jack. *Theatre in America, The Impact of Economic Forces, 1870–1967.* Ithaca: Cornell University Press, 1968.

Pollock, Thomas Clark. *Philadelphia Theatre in the 18th Century.* Philadelphia: University of Pennsylvania Press, 1933.

Pope-Hennessy, Dame Una. *Three Englishwomen in America.* London: Ernest Berwin, 1929.

Power-Waters, Alma. *John Barrymore, The Legend and the Man.* New York: Julian Messner, 1941.

Quinn, Arthur Hobson. "The Early Drama" *Cambridge History of American Literature.* Book Two, Chapter 2. New York: 1917.

_____. *A History of the American Drama from the Beginnings to the Civil War.* 2nd ed. New York: F.S. Crofts, 1943.

_____. *A History of the American Drama from the Civil War to the Present Day.* New York: F.S. Crofts, 1945.

Rankin, Hugh F. *Theatre in Colonial America.* Chapel Hill: University of North Carolina Press.

Reck, W. Emerson. *A. Lincoln: His Last 24 Hours.* Jefferson, N.C.: McFarland, 1987.

Rees, James. *The Dramatic Authors of America.* Philadelphia: G.B. Zieber, 1845.

Reignolds-Winslow, Catherine Mary (Kitty). *Yesterdays with Actors.* Boston: Cupples & Hurd, 1887.

Richardson, Charles F. *American Literature 1607-1885.* Vol. 2. New York: G. P. Putnam's Sons, 1891.

Rosenbach, Abraham Simon Wolfe. *The First Theatrical Company in America.* Worcester, Mass.: American Antiquarian Society, 1939.

Ruggles, Eleanor. *The Prince of Players, Edwin Booth.* New York: W.W. Norton, 1953.

Rushmore, Robert. *Fanny Kemble.* London: Crowell-Collier Press, Collier-Macmillan, 1970.

Rowson, Susanna Haswell. *Charlotte Temple.* F.W. Halsey, ed. New York, London: n.p., 1905.

————. *Charlotte Temple, A Tale of Truth — By Mrs. Rowson author of Victoria, Inquisitor, Fille de Chambre, etc.* Wilmington, Delaware: Printed by R. Porter, 1816. (This volume may be an undiscovered edition of the work since it is not listed in R.W.G. Vail's exhaustive bibliographical study of the printed works of Susanna Rowson. It is in the possession of the Wilmington Free Library Rare Books Collection.)

Rusk, Ralph Leslie. *The Literature of the Middle Western Frontier.* 2 Vols. New York: Frederick Ungar, 1925, 1953.

Sargent, Mary E. "Susanna Rowson" *Medford Historical Register.* April 7, 1904. pp. 24-40.

Schoberlin, Melvin H. *From Candles to Footlights.* With a preface by Barrett H. Clark. Denver: The Old West Publishing Co., 1941.

Seilhamer, George O. *A History of the American Theatre.* 3 Vols. Philadelphia: 1888-1891. Reissued by Haskell House. New York, 1969.

Sharp, Harold S., *Handbook of Pseudonyms & Personal Nicknames.* Vol. II. Metuchen, N.J.: Scarecrow, 1972.

Skinner, Otis. *Mad Folk of the Theatre.* Indianapolis: Bobbs-Merrill, 1928.

Smith, Sol. *The Theatrical Apprenticeship of Sol Smith.* N.p., n.d.

Snub, a citizen, (pseudonym). *A rub from Snub; or, a cursory analytical epistle addressed to Peter Porcupine ... containing glad tidings for the Democrats & a word of comfort to Mrs. S. Rowson, wherein the said porcupine's moral, political, critical, and literary character is fully illustrated.* Philadelphia: Printed for the Purchasers, 1795.

Sonneck, O.G. *Early Opera in America.* Reissued. New York: Benj. Blom, 1963.

Spargo, John. *Anthony Haswell, Printer, Patriot, Balladeer. A Biographical Study.* Rutlandt Vt.: Tuttle, 1925.

Stebbins, Emma. *Charlotte Cushman, Her Letters and Memories of Her Life.*

Boston: Houghton, Osgood. Cambridge, Mass.: Riverside, 1878.

Stone, Henry Dickinson. *Personal Recollections of the Drama, or, Theatrical Reminiscences.* N.p. 1873; reissued, New York, London: Benj. Blom, 1969.

Strang, Lewis Clinton. *Famous Actresses of the Day in America.* Vol. I. Boston: L.C. Page, 1899.

_____. *Famous Actresses of the Day in America.* 2nd Series. Boston: L.C. Page, 1902.

_____. *Famous Actors of the Day in America.* Boston: L.C. Page, 1900.

_____. *Players and Plays of the Last Quarter Century.* 2 vols. Boston: L.C. page, 1902.

Taubman, Howard. *The Making of American Theatre.* New York: Coward McCann, 1965.

Thomas, Lewis F., ed. *The Valley of the Mississippi.* Drawn and Lithographed by J.C. Wild. St. Louis: J.C. Wild, Chambers and Knapp Printers, 1841.

Towse, John Rankin. *Sixty Years of the Theatre.* New York: Funk & Wagnalls, 1916.

Trent, William Peterfield, John Erskine, Stuart P. Sherman and Carl Van Doren eds. *The Cambridge History of American Literature, Colonial and Revolutionary Literature; Early National Literature.* Vol. I. New York: G.P. Putnam's Sons, 1917.

Vail, Robert W.G. *Susanna Haswell Rowson; the Author of Charlotte Temple, a Bibliographical Study.* Worcester, Mass.: American Antiquarian Society. New Series. Vol. 42. 4/2/1932–10/19/1932. pp. 47–160.

Van Doren, Charles, ed. *Webster's American Biographical Dictionary.* New York: G. & C. Merriam, 1979.

Vaughn, Jack A. *Early American Dramatists from the Beginnings to 1900.* New York: Frederick Ungar, 1981.

Webster's Biographical Dictionary. Springfield, Mass.: G. & C. Merriam, 1972.

Wehrum, Victoria. *The American Theatre.* New York: Franklin Watts, 1974.

Weil, Dorothy. *In Defense of Women. Susanna Rowson 1762–1824.* University Park and London: The Pennsylvania State University Press, 1976.

Wemyss, Francis Courtney. *Theatrical Biographies of Eminent Actors & Authors.* New York: n.p., 1852.

_____. *Wemyss' Chronology of the American Stage from 1752–1852.* Reissued, New York: Benj. Blom, 1968.

_____. *Twenty-Six Years in the Life of an Actor & Manager.* 2 Vols. New York: n.p., 1847.

West, T. Hill, Jr. *The Theatre in Early Kentucky, 1790–1820.* Lexington: University Press of Kentucky, 1971.

Who Was Who in American History — Arts and Letters. Chicago: Marquis Who's Who, 1975.

Who Was Who in American History. 1607–1896. Revised ed. 1967. Chicago: Marquis Who's Who, 1963, 1967.

Wilson, Arthur H. *History of the Philadelphia Stage 1835–1855.* Philadelphia: n.p., 1935.

Wilson, Garff B. *History of American Acting.* Bloomington and London: Indiana University Press, 1966.

_____. *300 Years of American Drama and Theatre from "Ye Bare and Ye Cubb" to "Hair".* Englewood Cliffs, N.J.: Prentice-Hall, 1973.

Winter, William. *Brief Chronicles.* New York: Burt Franklin, 1970. 3 volumes in 1. A reprint of the 1889 edition originally published as Publications No. 7–8 and 10 of The Dunlap Society.

_____. *The Life and Art of Joseph Jefferson.* New York: Macmillan, 1894.

_____ *Other Days, Being Chronicles and Memories of the Stage.* New York: Moffatt Yard, 1908.

_____. *Shadows of the Stage.* 1st Series. New York: Macmillan, 1896.

_____. *Shadows of the Stage.* 2nd Series. Boston: Joseph Knight, 1893.

_____. *Vagrant Memories, Being Further Recollections of Other Days.* New York: Geo. H. Doran, 1915.

_____. *The Wallet of Time.* 2 Vols. New York: n.p., 1913.

Wood, William B. *Personal Recollections of the Philadelphia Stage,* Ed. by R.D. James, 1932. Philadelphia: n.p., 1855.

Woollcott, Alexander. *Mrs Fiske, Her Views on the Stage Recorded by Alexander Woollcott.* New York: Benj. Blom, reprint 1968, 1st Ed. 1917.

Wright, Constance. *Fanny Kemble and the Lovely Land.* New York: Dodd, Mead, 1972.

INDEX